Ultrasound in Assisted Reproduction and Early Pregnancy

Ultrasound in Assisted Reproduction and Early Pregnancy

A Practical Guide

Jane S. Fonda
University of Sydney

Rachael J. Rodgers
Royal Hospital for Women, Sydney

William L. Ledger
University of New South Wales

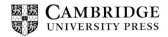

CAMBRIDGE
UNIVERSITY PRESS

University Printing House, Cambridge CB2 8BS, United Kingdom

One Liberty Plaza, 20th Floor, New York, NY 10006, USA

477 Williamstown Road, Port Melbourne, VIC 3207, Australia

314–321, 3rd Floor, Plot 3, Splendor Forum, Jasola District Centre, New Delhi – 110025, India

79 Anson Road, #06–04/06, Singapore 079906

Cambridge University Press is part of the University of Cambridge.

It furthers the University's mission by disseminating knowledge in the pursuit of education, learning, and research at the highest international levels of excellence.

www.cambridge.org
Information on this title: www.cambridge.org/9781108810210
DOI: 10.1017/9781108893794

First published 2021

Printed in Singapore by Markono Print Media Pte Ltd

A catalogue record for this publication is available from the British Library.

ISBN 978-1-108-81021-0 Paperback

Contents

Preface

Ultrasound imaging in gynaecology, as a diagnostic tool, has had a huge impact in patient management. It has been a privilege to be involved in medical imaging for my working career, and more recently, training nurses in gynaecology ultrasound specific to imaging required for patients in the field of assisted fertility. During the past 50 years there has been an unprecedented advance in technology. Ultrasound offers a non-ionising imaging modality and is the least expensive when compared to X-ray, nuclear medicine, CT and MRI.

Transvaginal ultrasound is an 'invasive' test, yet empathy and an ever-improving anatomical approach make it acceptable to patients. With the increased resolution it is able to visualise more clearly the detail of the structures and pathology if present. Where once it was performed in addition to a transabdominal scan, today it is more often the first-line approach.

This book was intended for the field of assisted fertility; however, it is also a text of ultrasound gynaecology and a guide for practitioners who use transvaginal ultrasound imaging of the female pelvis. The content is focused on gynaecology imaging and includes the most common appearances of normal, normal variants, physiological changes, pathology and induced changes seen during a stimulated menstrual cycle. Additional sections include early pregnancy, ultrasound procedures and technical advances.

My experience with ultrasound in fertility clinics began in the 1980s with transabdominal scanning. The development of the transvaginal probe and the 'focused' approach for imaging the uterus, the uterine endometrium and the ovaries to assess the number of follicles present have made sonography an integral part of patient monitoring, during menstrual cycles and assisted fertility treatments.

Trainee practitioners of sonography of the female pelvis come from diverse backgrounds, and sonography is a skill set with its various aspects to be learned. Writing this book has been enjoyable and rewarding and I hope that readers will find it useful.

Jane Fonda

Acknowledgements

My ultrasound career began in 1976, at the former St Margaret's Hospital in Darlinghurst. As a young radiographer, I enrolled in a sonography course, curious to explore the possibilities of this new technology. The matron, Sr Anne Byrne, RSJ, heard of my interest and offered me the opportunity to start the new ultrasound department. The newly designed 'Octoson' ultrasound machine, developed by the Ultrasonics Institute and made by the Australian company Ausonics Pty Ltd, was on order.

It was six months before the machine arrived. During this time, I was fortunate to learn this new modality at the Royal Hospital for Women (RHW), formerly in Paddington. Dr William Garrett, AO, director of the Imaging Department, and Dr Peter Warren and Kaye Griffiths, AO, from the Ultrasonics Institute (UI), became my mentors and I will be forever grateful to them for their guidance. Thanks to the association between the RHW and the former UI, with Dr George Kossoff as director, Dr David Robinson and the team gave me the opportunity to work on prototype machines, including the UI Octoson. The technical engineering was explained to me – many times – by Dr David Carpenter, Dr Jack Jellins, George Radovanovic and Ian Shepherd.

These early years were exciting times in the field of ultrasound. The Friday sessions at UI during which images were critiqued and artifacts characterised by the physicists added to my understanding and enabled me to improve the technical aspects of imaging. New clinical findings and technological developments were happening at an accelerated pace. Dr Rob Gill and Dr Michael Dadd introduced me to cardiac and Doppler imaging.

Lecturers, both local and from overseas, taught at the UI/RHW course, coordinated by Dr Laurie Wilson. I was asked to train the participants in the practical scanning sessions. Their enthusiasm for sonography impressed on me the importance of understanding normal anatomy before being able to appreciate anomalies.

For the next 40 plus years my career has introduced me to many colleagues and it is with fondness that I recall the doctors, sonographers, physicists, engineers, research scientists, technical staff and many others who developed my understanding and the practical considerations of ultrasound. With my experience in sonography and teaching I began my career as a lecturer at the University of Sydney in 1993, with Joanne (Murray) Lomas as course coordinator. The university provided me with many opportunities and encouraged me to obtain my master's in education. This book is a result of my years of teaching, many university lectures and presentations at scientific meetings and workshops in Australia and abroad.

I would like to thank Dr Fred Lomas for reading the first draft and suggesting it would be suitable for a wider field of gynaecology sonographers, Professor William Ledger for his enthusiastic response to my request for help in getting this book published and Dr Rachael Rodgers for her medical editing. I also thank my sonographer friends Adrienne Shepherd, Julie O'Brien, Rowena Gibson, Ellie Linton and Rosemary Gallagher, who assisted me with images. There are so many others who have shared their knowledge to whom I am truly grateful. On a more personal level, thanks to my children Melinda, Caroline, Martin and Emily for their encouragement and especially my husband Ben for his unfailing inspiration and support.

Introduction

Initially this book was conceived as an ultrasound imaging reference volume for nurses and clinicians working in the field of assisted reproductive technology (ART), to illustrate the use of ultrasound in fertility clinics. To reach a wider audience, more information was added, as a reference guide for trainee sonographers, medics, general gynaecologists and midwives.

Concomitant with use of sonography as a diagnostic imaging tool, it is equally important that the sonographer/practitioner have an inquisitive mind, as well as good spatial ability to understand relationships among physical objects. This book is intended to provide operators with an overview of the process and give a foundation to guide their ultrasound assessment of each individual and unique patient.

Sonography uses sound waves to produce a greyscale image of a slice (cross-sectional image) of a selected organ or combination of anatomical structures. In real time the cross-sectional images change with the movement of the probe. Very slight moves will change the view of the area being examined. Image acquisition during an ultrasound examination requires a steady hand and a keen eye.

The objective of ultrasound during a cycle of assisted conception is to identify the anatomic structures within the female pelvis, identify the uterus and measure the endometrium, identify both ovaries, count and measure the follicles and recognise and image pathology, if present. The examination can be extended, to include the kidneys or the peritoneal cavity for fluid.

Women should have had a comprehensive gynaecological scan prior to commencing assisted fertility treatment, ART; however, it is necessary to document any pathology identified, as it may be new or undetected on previous scans.

Ultrasound in ART provides visual monitoring of the endometrium of the uterus and the number and size of the follicles in the ovaries during the first part of the menstrual cycle. This visual record and the blood tests provide for a more accurate management plan to be used, for individual patient needs, whether she is on a monitored or medicated cycle.

Transvaginal ultrasound enables good resolution of the tissues in most cases; however, it is operator dependent. Knowledge of the relevant anatomy, physiology, physics and instrumentation and using a systematic approach are required to produce and interpret the images.

Pathology and congenital anomalies may also be seen during the examination. Some examples are also included in this text.

Transabdominal ultrasound may be required in cases in which the ovaries are located high in the pelvis and access is limited using the transvaginal approach.

Assisted conception procedures are designed to increase the chance of pregnancy. The treatments vary and depend on the cause of infertility.

Blood tests show the amount of oestrogen in the blood (serum oestradiol levels). On day seven or eight transvaginal ultrasound is performed to see how many follicles are developing in each ovary. With rising oestrogen levels, a repeat scan two days later will show further growth or maturity. Depending on the patient's response to treatment a third scan may be required.

When the follicles have reached an appropriate size, a medication is administered to trigger oocyte maturation and oocyte retrieval is planned.

The Role of Ultrasound in Fertility Treatments

The ultrasound appearance of the ovaries, during ovarian stimulation, differs dramatically with the growth of multiple follicles, compared to the ovaries in a natural cycle. In a stimulated cycle, follicle-stimulating hormone (FSH, with or without the addition of luteinising hormone [LH]) is administered, to encourage the growth of small follicles, to a size at which the collection of a mature oocytes becomes possible.

During the stimulation, either a gonadotropin-releasing hormone (GnRH) agonist or a GnRH antagonist is administered to prevent ovulation prior to the time of oocyte retrieval. If ovulation was to occur prior to the time of oocyte retrieval, the oocytes would be lost into the pelvis and retrieval would be extremely difficult.

The Natural Cycle

Ultrasound is performed on day 11–14 (approx.) to check the thickness of the endometrium. (Figure 1.1) A single dominant follicle is usually present on one ovary and several smaller follicles in each ovary. (Figure 1.2) The number of small follicles present in the ovaries will depend on the woman's ovarian reserve.

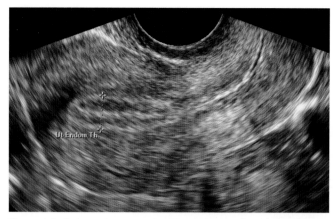

Figure 1.1 Endometrium measuring 10 mm, showing the tri-line appearance of the endometrium.

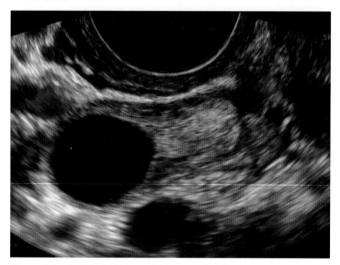

Figure 1.2 A single follicle seen in the natural cycle.

Ovulation Induction

Mild ovarian stimulation is conducted with medications such as clomiphene, letrozole or low-dose FSH to encourage the growth of one follicle. Ultrasound is used to check the number and size of follicles developing. If more than one follicle has developed, the cycle may be cancelled to avoid the potential of a multiple gestation.

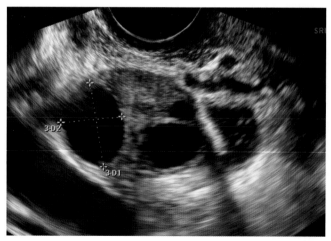

Figure 1.3 Right ovary with three follicles of various size seen in this one slice.

In Vitro Fertilisation Cycle

Ultrasound is used to check the number and size of the developing follicles within each ovary, during a stimulated cycle. Patients are monitored closely until the optimum number and size of developed follicles is reached.

With each scan, the endometrial lining of the uterus is assessed and measured in the mid to late proliferative phase. It grows under the influence of oestrogen during the ovary's follicular phase of the cycle.

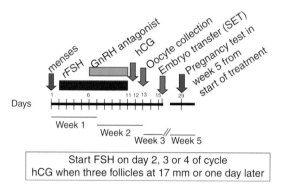

Start FSH on day 2, 3 or 4 of cycle
hCG when three follicles at 17 mm or one day later

Figure 1.4 Standard antagonist protocol. Reproduced with permission of W Ledger

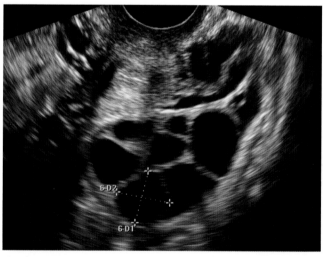

Figure 1.5 Multiple follicles in a stimulated in vitro fertilisation cycle.

Long Down-Regulation (Agonist)

The treatment cycle is a process of suppressing a woman's natural hormones before starting fertility medications.

Each woman should be independently evaluated to safely optimise egg quantity, without compromising quality. Long pituitary down-regulation protocols involve the administration of an agonist over four or more days before initiating ovarian stimulation.

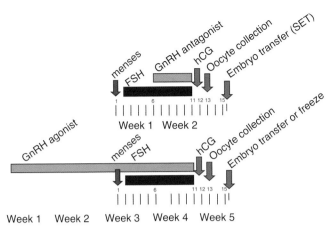

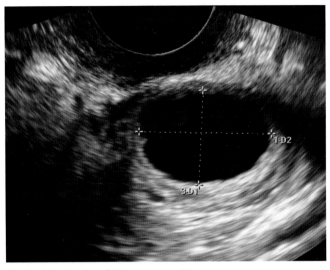

Figure 1.6 Agonist versus antagonist.
Reproduced with permission of W Ledger

Figure 1.8 Dominant follicle measuring 20 mm.

Anatomy and Physiology of the Female Reproductive System

The uterus and the ovaries are located deep in the female pelvis, between the urinary bladder and the rectum. The uterus measures approximately 7–8 cm in length and is a pear-shaped structure with the Fallopian tubes extending bilaterally from the cornua, the upper lateral aspects of the uterus. The uterus consists of the cervix, isthmus, body and fundus. The muscle wall of the uterus is the myometrium and the inner lining of the body of the uterus is the endometrium.

The inner endometrial layer is the functional layer into which the embryo implants. It increases in thickness during the menstrual cycle and is shed during menstruation if conception does not occur. Figure 1.9

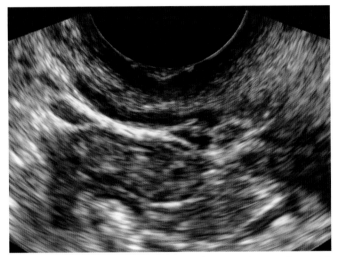

Figure 1.7 Agonist cycle before the start of fertility medications show small follicles in the ovary located between the uterus to the right of image, the pelvic wall to the left and bowel seen deep to the ovary.

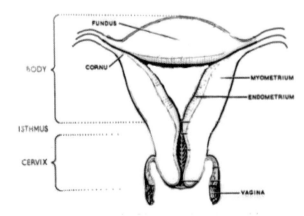

Figure 1.9 Coronal section of the uterus.

Scan Prior to Embryo Transfer

The timing for thawed embryos to be transferred depends on tracking the ovarian cycle. Prior to the embryo transfer, ultrasound is used to determine the thickness of the endometrium and to assess each ovary, looking for a dominant follicle, in a natural cycle, and an absence of large follicles in a medicated cycle.

This scan, with the blood test results, is for the purpose of determining the optimal time to be planned for the fertilised ovum to be transferred to the uterine cavity. see Figures 1.1 and 1.8

The parietal peritoneum is the lining of the abdominal cavity, which extends from the anterior wall into the pelvis, to cover the superior wall of the bladder and folds back on itself, at the level of the uterine isthmus to cover the anterior body of the uterus. Passing over the fundus, it extends over the posterior body of the uterus to the level of the cervix and folds upwards to cover the rectum, forming the recto-uterine pouch or pouch of Douglas (POD). Accumulated free fluid in the peritoneal cavity may be seen in the POD.

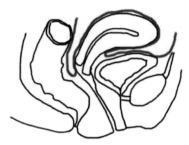

Figure 1.10 Folds of the peritoneum seen in median sagittal section of the female pelvis.

A double peritoneal fold forms the broad ligament of the uterus and extends laterally, from the uterus to the side walls and floor of the pelvis. The broad ligament encases the Fallopian tubes, within a small mesentery called the mesosalpinx. The ovarian and uterine blood vessels, lymphatics and nerves pass within the suspensory ligament of the ovary, which becomes continuous with the mesovarium of the broad ligament.

The uterine arteries arise on each side from the anterior branch of the iliac arteries. They pass anterior to the ureter to the uterus, in the cardinal ligament, through the inferior broad ligament and up along the lateral walls of the uterus to connect (anastomose) with the ovarian arteries.

The ovaries are located on the posterior aspect of the broad ligament, suspended by ovarian mesothelium. The ovaries are attached to the ligament by the utero-ovarian ligaments. Each ovary measures approximately $30 \times 20 \times 10$ mm. The ovaries are not covered by peritoneum and the oocyte expelled at ovulation passes into the peritoneal cavity and is trapped by the fimbriae of the infundibulum of the uterine tube and carried into the ampulla, where it may be fertilised.

The cervix protrudes into the upper vagina, and the recess around the cervix is the vaginal fornix. The recess behind the cervix is called the posterior fornix. The smaller recesses anterior and laterally are the anterior and lateral fornices. The transvaginal probe is directed into this space to image the uterus and ovaries.

The uterine cavity is continuous with the cervical canal, which passes through the isthmus, the body of the uterus and laterally into each Fallopian tube. The distal fimbrial end of each fallopian tube opens into the peritoneal cavity and lies in close proximity to the ovary.

Uterine Position

The cervix is located centrally in the pelvis, being supported anteriorly by the pubo-cervical ligament, laterally by the transverse cervical or cardinal ligament and posteriorly by the uterosacral ligament.

Uterine position within the pelvis can vary from anteverted, where the fundus is anterior to the cervix, to retroverted, with the fundus located posterior to the cervix, also anteflexed and retroflexed.

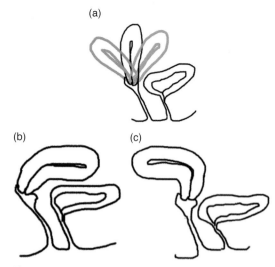

Figure 1.11 (a) The uterine position is described as anteverted (blue), retroverted (green), or in the long axis (black) by the position of the fundus being anterior, posterior or in line with the cervix. (b, c) The uterus seen in anteflexed and retroflexed position.

The Menstrual Cycle

The hormonal control of the menstrual cycle is complex. It is regulated by the hypothalamic–pituitary–ovarian axis. The hypothalamus releases GnRH in a pulsatile manner. This stimulates the anterior pituitary to release FSH and LH. FSH stimulates the growth of ovarian follicles. Around day 14 of a 28-day menstrual cycle, rising oestrogen levels trigger a surge of LH to be released from the anterior pituitary. The LH surge triggers the maturation of the oocyte contained in the dominant follicle. Approximately 36–38 hours after the LH surge, ovulation occurs.

Following ovulation, the theca granulosa cells of the follicle transform into lutein cells, and the follicle becomes known as the corpus luteum. If pregnancy does not occur, the corpus luteum ceases production of progesterone. The sudden drop in serum progesterone triggers menstruation.

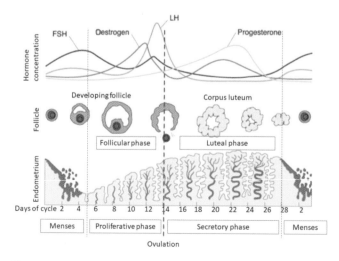

Figure 1.12 Menstrual cycle.
Reproduced with permission of W Ledger

Physiology of the Uterus

Throughout the menstrual cycle, the endometrium thickens and the change in appearance can be seen and measured using ultrasound. Measurements are taken through both layers from the basal layer to the opposite basal layer, reaching a maximum diameter of 14 mm during the secretory phase of the cycle.

The uterus is a dynamic organ, and with real-time ultrasound imaging contractions may be seen in midcycle. A slow wave moves along the endometrium from the internal os towards the fundus.

After menses the endometrium is seen as a thin line, which thickens during the proliferative phase of the cycle.

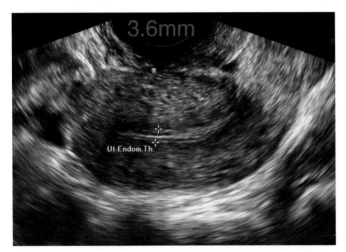

Figure 1.13 Endometrium is thin: day 5 of the cycle.

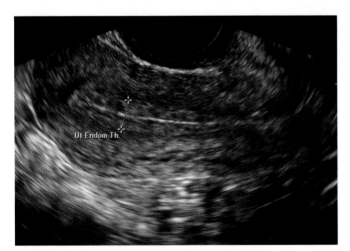

Figure 1.14 Endometrial thickness has increased to 6.8 mm but the basal layer is not echogenic.

By day 10 of the cycle the endometrium will be seen with the echogenic basal layer surrounding the endometrium with the uterine cavity in the centre, creating the tri-line appearance.

The endometrium measurement is taken, in the image of the long axis of the uterus, from the outer edge of the basal layer to the outer edge of the basal layer on the opposite side, at 90 degrees to the cavity echo. Optimal measurements in the late proliferative phase are 7–12 mm.

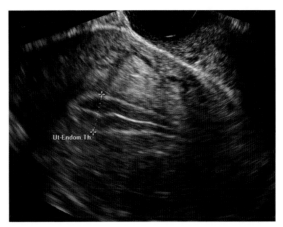

Figure 1.15 Endometrium with tri-line appearance caused by the echogenic basal layer surrounding the echogenic central cavity layer. These surfaces are at 90 degrees to the beam and act as specular reflectors.

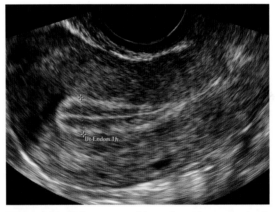

Figure 1.16 Tri-line pattern of the endometrium measuring 9 mm.

After ovulation, in the secretory phase of the cycle, the endometrium is seen on ultrasound as being echogenic, due to the many reflections from the surfaces of the more tortuous vessels. The maximum full thickness of the endometrium is 14 mm at days 19–23.

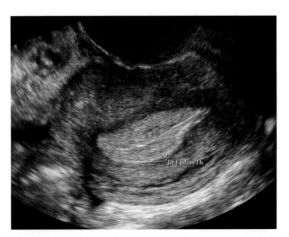

Figure 1.17 Ultrasound appearance of the endometrium in the secretory phase of the menstrual cycle. The increase in echogenicity is due to the increase in the number and tortuosity of the reflecting surfaces of vessels and glands within the endometrium.

Physiology of the Ovaries

Changes within the ovaries occur during the menstrual cycle, with the growth of follicles, ovulation and the development of the corpus luteum after ovulation.

Follicles in the ovary can be visualised on ultrasound as fluid-filled structures, physiological cysts.

In women who do not have a reduced ovarian reserve, several small follicles can be seen in each ovary during the first half of the menstrual cycle (follicular phase). In women with a reduced ovarian reserve (most commonly older women), these small follicles may not be present.

The lead or dominant follicle will accelerate in growth, from about day 10 to produce a follicle approximately 20 mm in diameter, by approximately day 13 of a 28-day menstrual cycle.

Ovulation will occur shortly afterwards. The oocyte is located on the wall of the follicle, within a cluster of cumulus cells, and is too small to be seen with ultrasound. The follicle becomes the corpus luteum after ovulation.

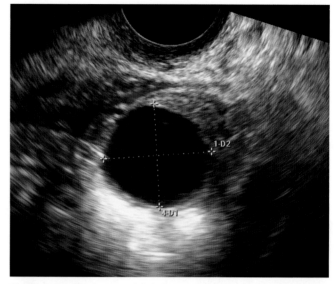

Figure 1.19 The dominant follicle is 24 mm, which will produce a mature ovum.

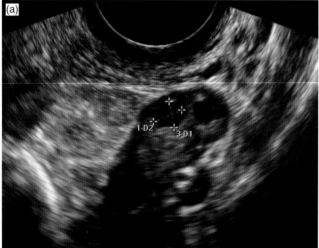

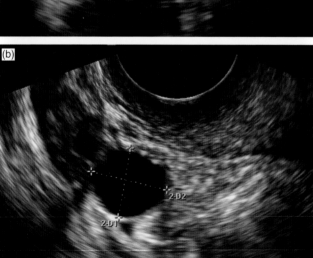

Figure 1.18 (a, b) The left and right ovaries in an unstimulated menstrual cycle. The left ovary contains three small follicles <7 mm and on the right is the developing dominant follicle of 14 mm.

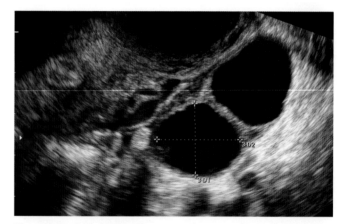

Figure 1.20 Stimulated ovaries may produce more than one mature ovum.

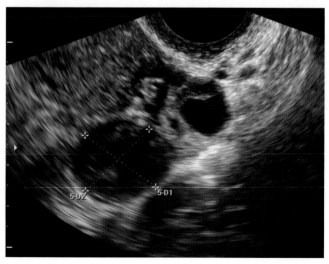

Figure 1.21 Corpus luteum forms post ovulation in the luteal phase of the menstrual cycle.

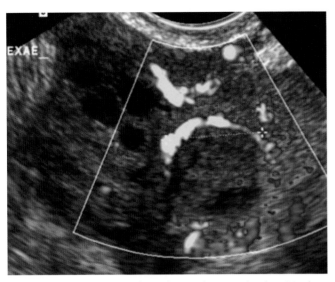

Figure 1.22 Corpus luteum shows the vascular ring with colour Doppler.

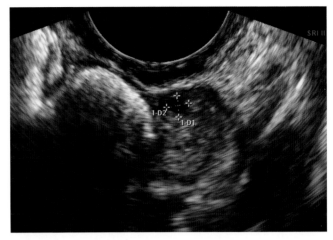

Figure 1.24 Unstimulated ovary.

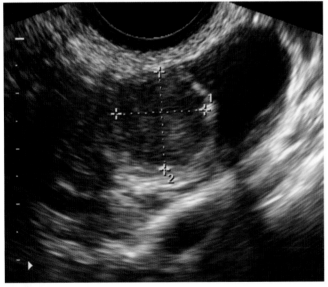

Figure 1.23 Corpus luteum, haemorrhagic cyst and endometrioma may have a similar appearance on ultrasound.

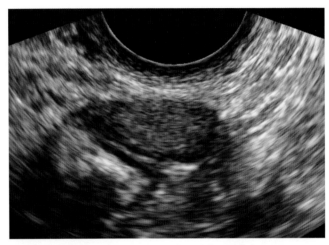

Figure 1.25 Perimenopausal ovary with no defined follicles.

Fluid in the Pelvis

A full bladder is not required for a transvaginal scan. If the bladder is partially filled it is seen as an anechoic structure anterior to the uterus. Figure 1.26

Free fluid may be seen as an anechoic collection in the POD or around the ovaries. The anechoic fluid collection will fill the space between the anatomical structures within the pelvis.

Small pockets of physiological free fluid may be seen in the pelvis.

A small amount of free fluid may be seen at any time during the menstrual cycle and is considered normal in asymptomatic premenopausal women. Figures 1.27, 1.28

Large pockets of free fluid may be due to infection or other medical conditions.

Ovarian hyperstimulation syndrome results in the ultrasound appearance of enlarged ovaries with multiple follicles and free fluid in the pelvis extending into the abdomen and in severe cases in the chest cavity. Figures 1.30, 1.31

Perimenopausal Ovaries

Ovaries may be difficult to see in the perimenopausal or post-menopausal patient, due to the lack of follicles. The ovarian tissue is identified by location, medial to the iliac vessels and lateral to the uterus and its hypoechoic appearance compared to the surrounding structures. Look closely for small (<3 mm) cysts within the ovary. Figures 1.24 and 1.25

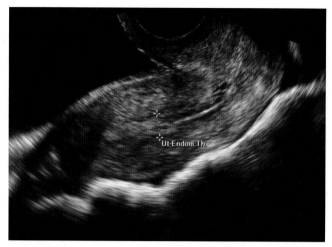

Figure 1.26 Transvaginal scan with a full bladder anterior to the uterus and a physiological small collection posterior to the uterus and in the pouch of Douglas.

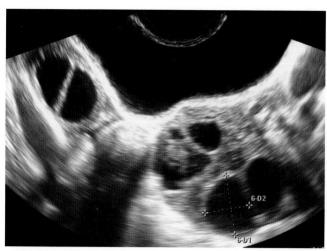

Figure 1.29 The ovaries scanned through the full bladder in this transvaginal study.

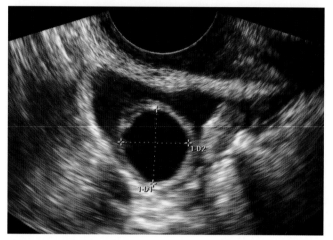

Figure 1.27 Pocket of free fluid around a single ovarian follicle.

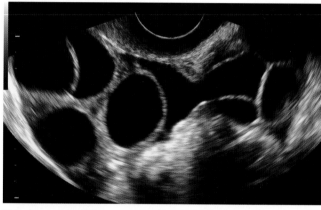

Figure 1.30 Free fluid seen between the right and left ovaries.

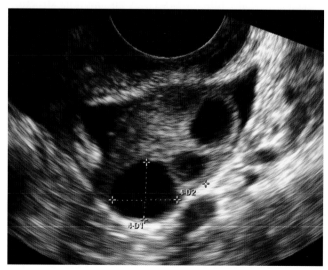

Figure 1.28 The fluid is seen adjacent to the outline of the ovary between the pelvic wall laterally and the uterus medially.

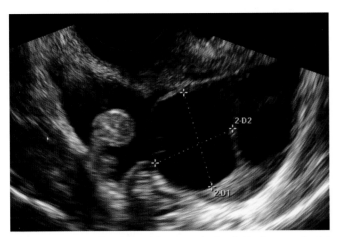

Figure 1.31 Loop of small bowel floating in the free fluid adjacent to the right ovary.

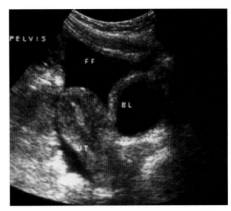

Figure 1.32 Transabdominal scan of the pelvis showing free fluid in excess of 300 ml.

Transabdominal scanning is required to assess large amounts of free fluid in the abdomen. Use the transabdominal approach to investigate the extent of the fluid in the upper abdomen, including Morrison's pouch and above the diaphragm. Figure 1.32

Physics and Instrumentation

Ultrasound Machine

The ultrasound machine console varies between companies in the layout of the knobs. However, the overall panels are very similar, labelled and become familiar with use.

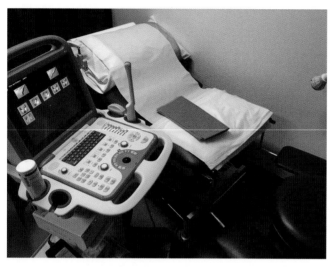

Figure 2.1 Position of the bed, chair and machine console are adjusted for individual sonographer comfort.

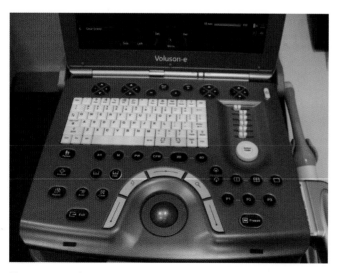

Figure 2.2 Machine console.

Basic Scanning Protocol

Ultrasound machines vary in the actual layout of the console. The settings most often used for greyscale imaging are

1. **New Patient**: will remove all previous data acquired in a previous examination
2. **Depth**: adjusted as required to optimise the area being examined
3. **Focus**: positioned at or just posterior to the area of interest
4. **Gain**: adjusted to balance the overall greyscale of the image
5. **Time gain compensation (TGC)**: adjusts the level of greyscale to be uniform from superficial to deep
6. **Freeze**: to capture the best image on the screen
7. **Callipers**: to measure the thickness of the endometrium and follicles
8. **Print**: to store the image

The machine is cleaned and prepared using the ON/OFF button to activate and NEW PATIENT to enter data and ensure previous patient data are deleted. Select the TRANSDUCER and the STUDY (gynaecology). Factory settings for the study will be activated, which include depth, gain, TGC, focal depth, annotation, and measurement settings. These settings can be altered according to the appearance of the image on the screen. The FREEZE button is activated so the image will appear in real time on the screen.

Transducers designed for transvaginal scanning provide good tissue definition. Allow sufficient depth in the field of view to locate the structures and then adjust the depth to optimise the required image. Figure 2.3

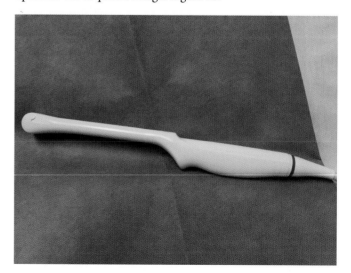

Figure 2.3 Transvaginal probe.

Physics of Ultrasound

The physics of ultrasound is important; however, a comprehensive discussion will not be covered in this text. For the practitioner, selecting the appropriate transducer and understanding the console to select the appropriate preset and controls to optimise image resolution are required. Developing the skill in spatial relationships, to manipulate the probe to provide the best acoustic window and to assess anatomy in greyscale imaging, comes with practice.

The ability to recognise artifacts and the limitations of ultrasound develops over time. Sonography is a new skill and requires supervision to start and independent competence with practice.

The following is a brief outline of how the image is produced, using high-frequency sound waves passing through tissue, with the image produced by the reflected echoes, from various interfaces, of the different tissues.

The ultrasound machine is composed of a computer hard drive, transducer, console, keyboard, monitor and printer or storage system. The software in modern machines is preprogrammed to suit each examination; however, adjustments can be made to maximise the image quality. The clarity of the image is essential for the accurate placement of callipers for measurements. New technology using silicon chips is advancing image quality.

Transducers are designed to optimise imaging of specific areas. Within the transducer is an array of piezoelectric crystal elements. The diagnostic ultrasound frequency range is 2–15 million Hertz or 2–15 MHz. The pulse length is frequency dependent. A higher frequency transducer will provide better resolution; however, it the beam will not penetrate as far as with lower frequency transducers. Abdominal transducers are 2–5 MHz, transvaginal transducers are 5–10 MHz, while transducers designed for superficial structures are in the 7–15 MHz range approximately.

The pulse-echo principle describes how the image is generated, as follows: (1) The electrical pulse strikes the crystal, which vibrates. (2) The produced sound beam propagates through tissue. (3) Echoes arising from tissue interfaces are reflected back to the crystal. (4) The crystal vibrates, generating an electrical impulse.

Each crystal element within the transducer sends out a pulse and receives echoes along the same line of sight, and the depth of each echo is related to the time from pulse transmitted to echo received. The image is composed of multiple lines from the array of crystals within the transducer.

As the pulse passes through the tissues of the body, echoes are generated by the many interfaces and scatterers. Echoes are reflected from interfaces of tissues with different acoustic impedance. Some energy is reflected back to the transducer, while the remainder is transmitted into the second medium. Interfaces with very large acoustic impedance difference, that is, soft tissue and air or soft tissue and bone, create a barrier and all of the energy is reflected and none is transmitted into the second tissue. The speed of sound in human tissues and liquids is determined by their density and stiffness, average 1540 m/s.

Resolution is the ability to distinguish echoes in terms of space, time and strength, and good resolution is critical to the production of high-quality images. Resolution is determined by the frequency of the transducer in the axial plane and the beam width in the lateral plane. Beam width artifact is caused by divergence of the beam in the far field deep to the focal zone.

Acoustic windows are areas of the patient through which the ultrasound beam can pass to visualise deeper structures. When the organ is located the probe is slowly moved to study the structures and produce the best image. Examine organs in longitudinal, transverse and oblique planes to assess size, shape, margins and echogenicity.

Greyscale imaging in ultrasound is a cross-sectional image of a slice of the body, with a limited depth. The range is from white through shades of grey to black. Strong reflectors are white, echogenic. Fluid, that is, urine, bile, blood or fluid within a cyst, is black, anechoic. Soft tissue is demonstrated in shades of grey. The sound wave will be totally reflected at a tissue/air and tissue/bone interface.

The GAIN button on the console can be adjusted to make the image darker or brighter. The TGC sliders will adjust the greyscale of the image in the near field to the far field. Even shades of grey should be seen superficially and at depth.

Echogenicity is a term used in ultrasound to describe the shades of grey. Lighter shades are more echogenic (hyperechoic) and darker ones less echogenic (hypoechoic), while black is anechoic. Complex mass refers to a structure having both solid and cystic components and is described as predominantly solid or cystic.

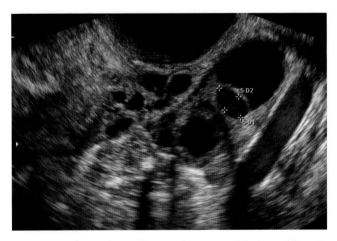

Figure 2.4 Left ovary located between the uterus and the internal iliac vein. Greyscale imaging defines the outline of the ovary and the cluster of arcuate vessels of the uterus.

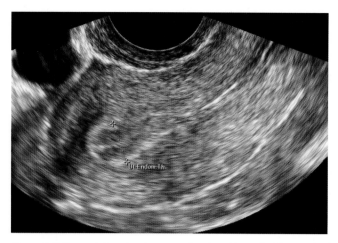

Figure 2.5 Greyscale imaging demonstrating the white outline (hyperechoic) of the uterus and the endometrium.

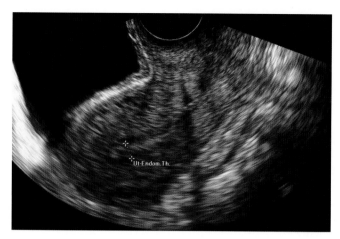

Figure 2.6 The full bladder is pushing the uterus away from the optimal plane of 90 degrees, making the endometrium less well defined.

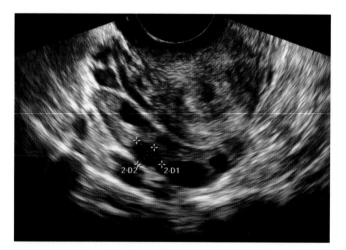

Figure 2.7 Greyscale imaging shows the ovary, with anechoic follicles, located in the pouch of Douglas posterior to the cervix. The margin between the cervix and ovary is the hyperechoic line.

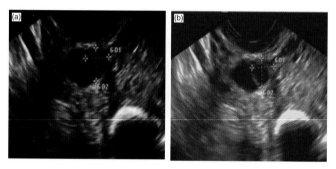

Figure 2.8 Gain setting needed to be increased to visualise the membrane between the two small follicles.

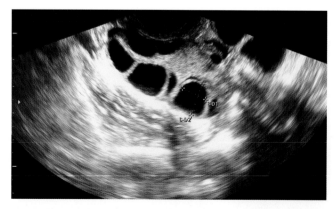

Figure 2.9 Overall gain setting is too high, and the image brighter white than required, diminishing the contrast between the ovary and the bowel.

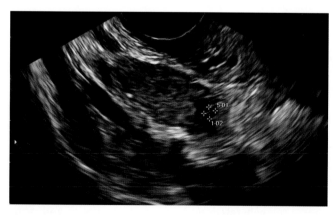

Figure 2.10 Unstimulated ovary is hypoechoic compared to the surrounding structures. A small follicle is measured.

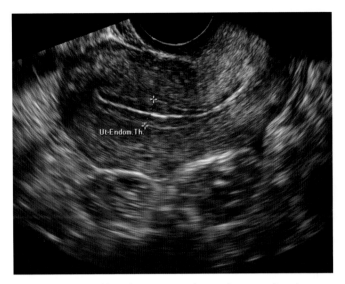

Figure 2.11 Normal bowel pattern seen deep to the uterus. Bowel patterns vary due to content; however, peristalsis will be seen with real-time imaging.

Acoustic Artifacts

There are multiple ways that artifacts are produced in images using ultrasound. This brief discussion will cover enhancement, shadowing, comet tail, ringdown, beam width and side lobe artifacts, commonly seen with transvaginal scanning.

Enhancement

Enhancement is seen behind a non-attenuating structure. There is no attenuation through a fluid-filled cyst and the area directly deep to the cyst will appear whiter (enhanced) than the adjacent tissue (Figure 2.14).

Characteristics of a **simple cyst** are

- Rounded thin wall structure
- Fluid filled (black)
- No internal echoes
- Acoustic enhancement posterior (Gill, 2012, pp. 53–69)

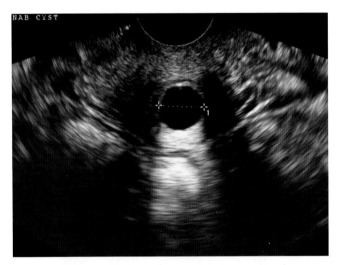

Figure 2.14 Acoustic enhancement deep to a fluid-filled cyst.

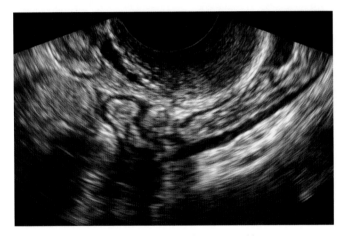

Figure 2.12 Bowel wall muscle is hypoechoic. Mucosal layer is more echogenic. Content of the bowel will create a variety of appearances. Peristalsis can be observed in real-time imaging.

With the increase in the fluid content of the blood vessels and glands, in the endometrial lining, posterior enhancement may be seen in the myometrium.

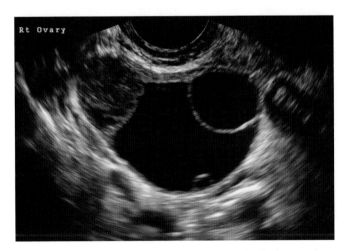

Figure 2.13 Haemorrhagic cyst with hypoechoic low-level echoes, and two anechoic follicles, within the right ovary.

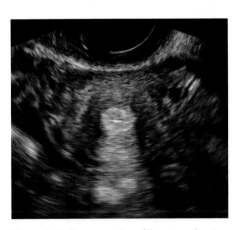

Figure 2.15 Transverse view of the uterus showing acoustic enhancement in the myometrium, deep to the less attenuating endometrium.

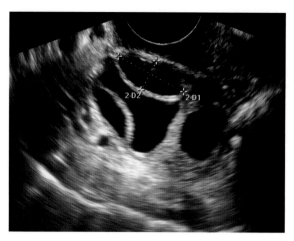

Figure 2.16 The acoustic enhancement is blended with the hyperechoic echoes behind or deep to the ovary.

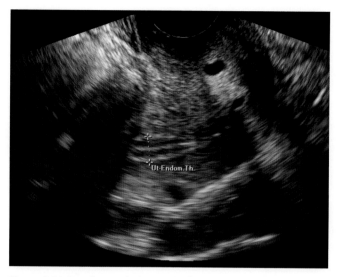

Figure 2.19 Bowel gas is shadowing the fundus of the uterus.

Shadowing

Multiple artifacts are produced by the sound beam passing through tissue. An **acoustic shadow** is produced behind a strong reflecting interface or strong attenuating tissue. The interface between soft tissue and air, bone or calcified structures will produce shadowing, posteriorly.

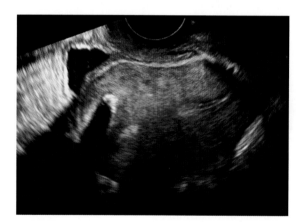

Figure 2.17 Acoustic shadowing deep to calcification of a uterine fibroid.

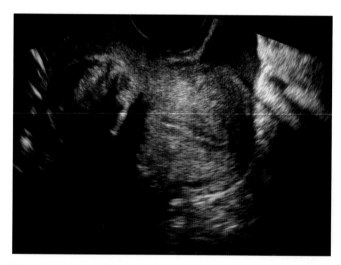

Figure 2.20 Uterine fibroid with irregular density causing acoustic shadowing.

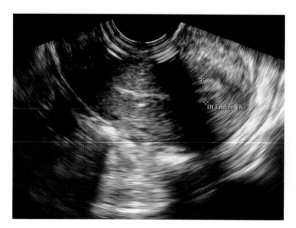

Figure 2.18 Acoustic shadowing caused by air between the condom and the transducer.

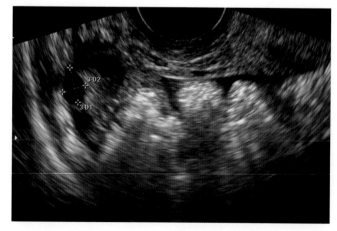

Figure 2.21 Acoustic shadow. Gas in bowel, seen medial to the right ovary, as bright white echoes. Loops of bowel are imaged here in cross section. Posterior to the gas are white 'comet tail' artifacts, referred to as 'dirty shadowing'. If the ovary is located posterior to the bowel it will not be seen.

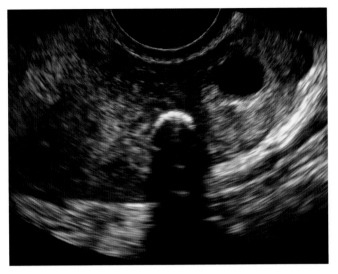

Figure 2.22 Shadowing behind a calcified fibroid. Note how the surface of the fibroid prevents penetration of the beam. Also seen is an anechoic Nabothian cyst with slight posterior enhancement.

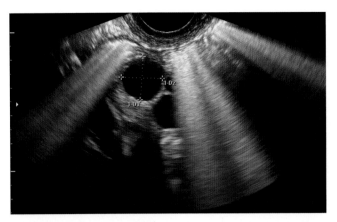

Figure 2.24 Gas in the bowel has created a resonance (ringdown) artifact, which prevents visualisation of the structures deep to the gas.

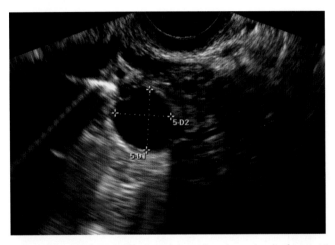

Figure 2.25 Ringdown artifact seen deep to the echogenic echo from gas in the bowel, to the left of the follicle.

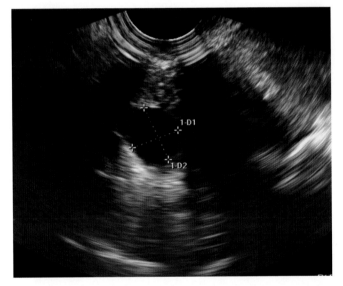

Figure 2.23 Loss of contact between the transducer and the tissue produces shadowing.

Ringdown Artifact

Ringdown artifacts are a result of resonance, induced by the ultrasound beam, when it strikes multiple air bubbles and is trapped between two strong parallel reflectors. The high reflectivity of the gas interfaces produces a stream of bright echoes, which extends from the source into deeper structures (Gent, 2012, p. 204).

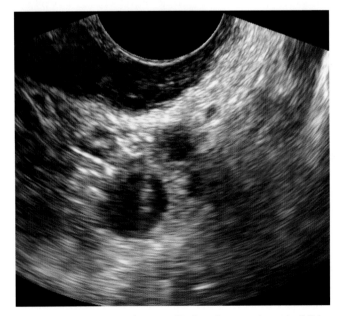

Figure 2.26 Ringdown artifact caused by bowel gas anterior to the follicle producing the echogenic line through the anechoic follicle, mimicking a membrane. Fan the beam and the artifact will move across the follicle.

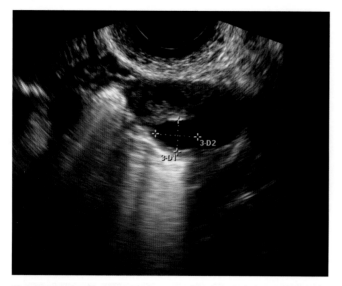

Figure 2.27 Gas-filled bowel is the cause of the hyperechoic ringdown artifact medial and deep to the left ovary.

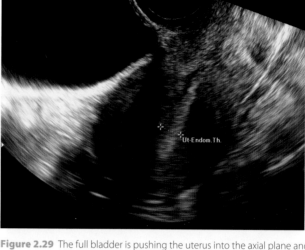

Figure 2.29 The full bladder is pushing the uterus into the axial plane and the endometrium appears echogenic with the margin not well defined due to beam width artifact, which is also seen on the posterior bladder wall.

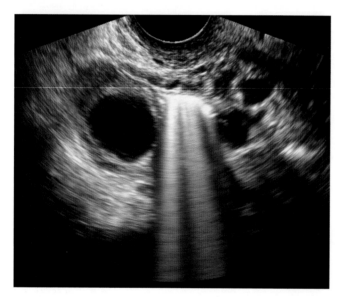

Figure 2.28 Ringdown artifact.

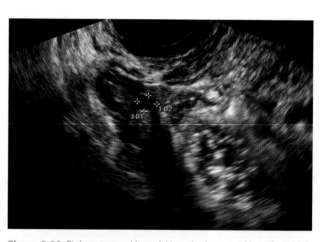

Figure 2.30 Right ovary and bowel. Note the beam width artifacts in the bowel echoes at depth.

Beam Width Artifact

Beam width artifact causes the echoes to be written as a line, perpendicular to the beam, rather than a dot at depth. This is caused by divergence of the beam, deep to the focal zone. Figures 2.29

Ultrasound image interpretation in gynaecology is based on an understanding of anatomy and physiology. Each image represents a single slice of tissue. With real-time imaging and an understanding of the clinical history, the 3D interpretation is collated mentally, by moving the probe through the area or the organ being investigated.

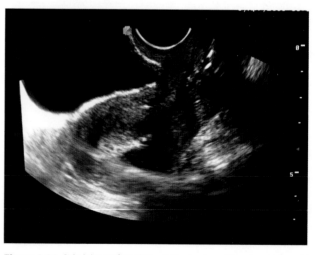

Figure 2.31 Side-lobe artifact, through the fundus of the uterus, caused by reflections from the distal bladder wall but placed in the field of view. This band of echoes will move independent of the uterus when the probe is moved forward or withdrawn slightly, showing it to be artifact and not the uterine echoes.

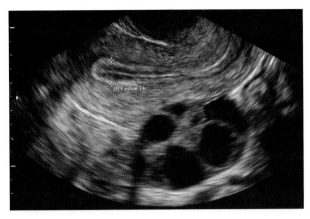

Figure 2.32 The uterus provides an acoustic window to see the ovary located in the pouch of Douglas.

Colour Doppler Imaging

Colour Doppler is used in ultrasound to demonstrate flow in blood vessels. It is obtained by measurement of movement of the red blood cells. These signals can then be colour coded, which allows blood vessels to be identified and adds clarity to the study. Figures 2.33, 2.34, 2.35, 2.36, 2.37, 2.38, 2.39a, 2.39b, 2.40

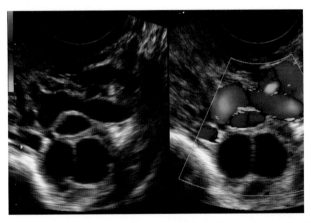

Figure 2.33 Colour Doppler demonstrates blood flow in the vessels adjacent to the ovary.

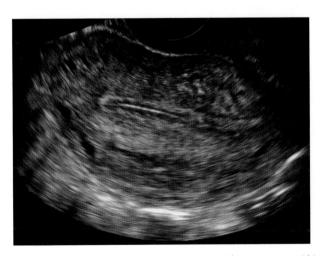

Figure 2.34 Arcuate blood vessels are seen as anechoic structures within the outer wall of the uterus.

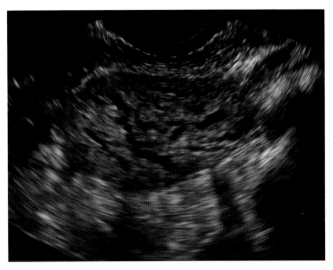

Figure 2.35 Arcuate blood vessels are seen as anechoic structures in this long axis view of the lateral uterine wall.

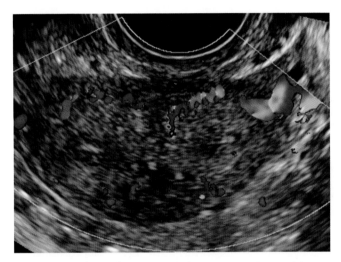

Figure 2.36 Colour perfusion is seen in the arcuate vessels around the outer uterine wall in the transverse view of the fundus of a bicornuate uterus.

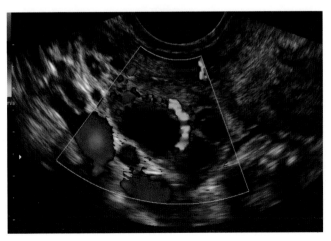

Figure 2.37 Corpus luteum is seen with a highly vascular ring of vessels.

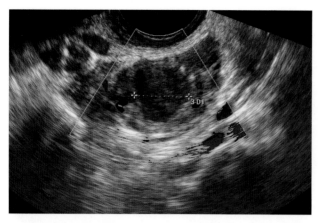

Figure 2.38 Haemorrhagic cysts contain low-level echoes with no evidence of blood flow within.

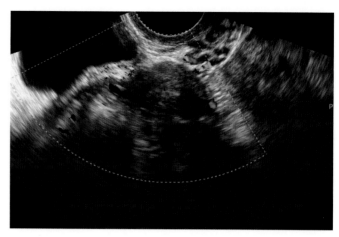

Figure 2.40 Colour Doppler may be helpful to locate a non-stimulated ovary.

(a)

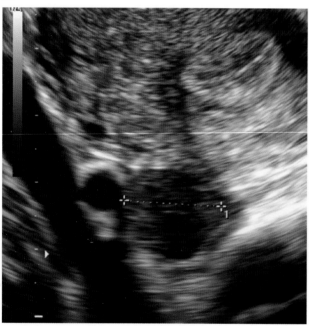

(b)

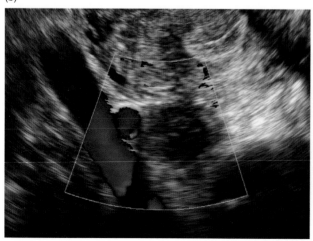

Figure 2.39 (a) Right ovary next to blood vessel. (b) Colour Doppler is used to distinguish a blood vessel next to the right ovary seen in (a).

3D/4D Ultrasound Imaging

3D ultrasound is volume rendering of the ultrasound data and presents an image with depth perspective. Volumetric probes produce volume-rendered images in real time or 4D imaging (three spatial dimensions plus one time dimension). The data can be stored and reviewed in several planes.

It is imperative to obtain good B-mode (2D black and white) imaging to assess the area for the volume acquisition.

The greyscale in the 2D image needs to be carefully managed to obtain good texture in the volume image. Image reconstruction requires more complex equipment than for 2D imaging. Figures 2.41, 2.42

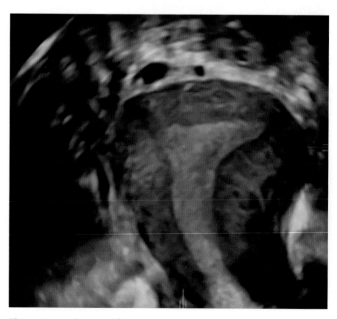

Figure 2.41 3D image of the uterus and endometrium. Courtesy of E Linton Kogarah Medical Imaging

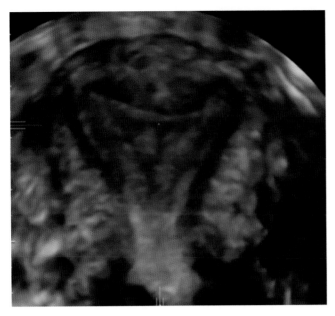

Figure 2.42 3D image of arcuate uterus.
Courtesy of E Linton Kogarah Medical Imaging

3D Colour Imaging

Further advances in ultrasound equipment have specialised software designed to automatically calculate the number and volume of follicles, from a 3D ovarian volume, with 3D colour imaging. Figures 2.43, 2.44

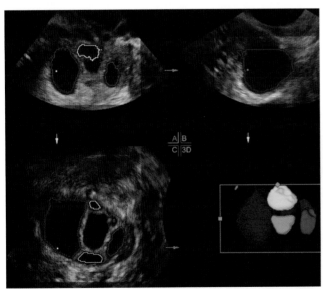

Figure 2.43 3D colour image of follicles.

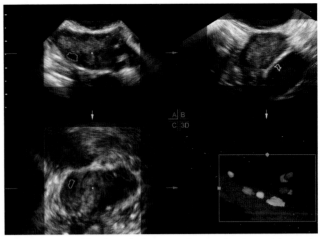

Figure 2.44 The blood vessel adjacent to the ovary has been picked up in the volume image. This can be subtracted prior to reporting.

Scanning Protocol

The room for each examination should be prepared and clean and have all supplies within easy reach.

Check each patient's full name and date of birth.

Although the patients are usually familiar with TV imaging, briefly explain the examination and obtain their consent to proceed with the examination.

Check that the patient does not have an allergy to Latex. If so, then use Latex-free probe covers.

Sonographers wear gloves for transvaginal scanning. Latex-free gloves are available. Hands are washed between patients.

Real-time imaging allows us to

- Identify major anatomic structures seen in the female pelvis with ultrasound.
- Identify changes seen on ultrasound imaging throughout the menstrual cycle.
- Measure the thickness of the endometrium.
- Count and measure each follicle in both ovaries
- Identify pathology. It is so important to know the appearance of normal anatomy first, to be able to recognise variations from normal and identify anomalies.

Transvaginal Imaging

Gel is applied to the transvaginal transducer (probe) and it is covered with a probe cover. It is important to ensure there are no air bubbles between the transducer and the probe cover, as the air will block the transmission of the sound waves into the tissue. Gel is applied again to the tip of the covered probe. Saline can also be used to lubricate.

Tips for Scanning

- Position the probe to image the structure.
- Adjust the angle to optimise the tissue plane.
- Adjust **depth** to include the whole structure.
- Adjust **focus** marker(s) to level of interest.
- **TGC:** balance greyscale (near and far fields).
- **Gain:** overall greyscale
- **Dynamic range** is decreased to enhance margins.
- Move through each organ to check

  Size

  Shape

  Echotexture

  Margins

  Internal architecture

(a)

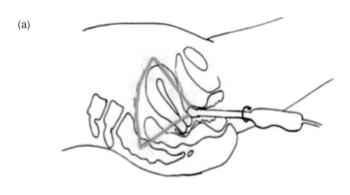

(b)

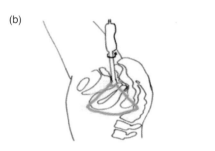

Figure 2.46 (a) The actual orientation of the probe and the patient position. (b) The orientation of the image as seen on the screen.

The image seen on the monitor displays the transducer at the top of the screen. Transvaginally, in the sagittal plane the anterior aspect of the pelvis is to the left of the image and the posterior aspect is to the right of the image seen on the monitor screen. The vertical mirror image can also be used; however, this is the orientation of most practices in Australia.

(a)

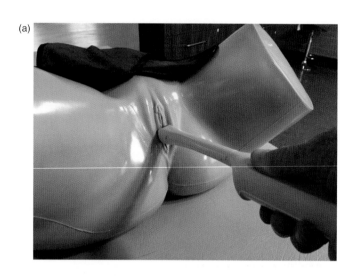

(b)

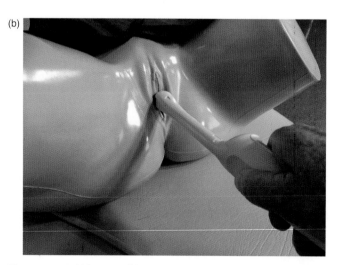

Figure 2.45 (a, b) Position of the transvaginal probe in the long axis and short axis. Note the position of the thumb on the probe handle. Rotate the probe counter-clockwise from the 12 o'clock sagittal to 9 o'clock coronal plane.

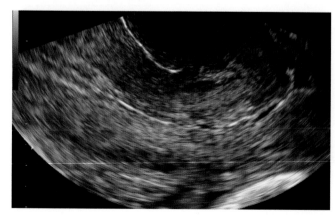

Figure 2.47 Long axis view of uterine cervix.

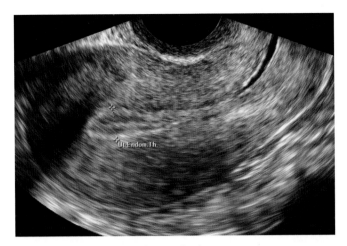

Figure 2.48 Long axis view of uterine fundus.

In the transverse plane of the uterus, the image is displayed with the right side of the patient to the left of the screen. Angling the probe from the cervix, sweeping through to the fundus in the transverse plane of the uterus demonstrates anomalies such as bicornuate or subseptate uterus.

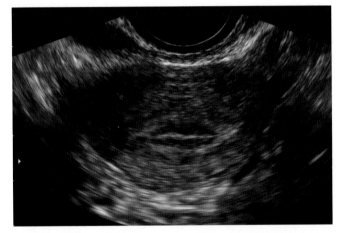

Figure 2.49 Transverse view showing normal appearance of the uterus.

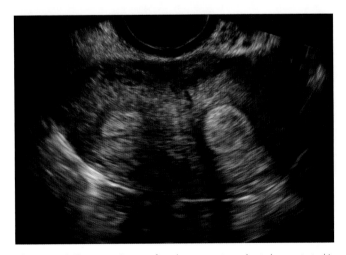

Figure 2.50 Transverse image of a subseptate uterus, best demonstrated in the transverse plane.

Move the probe from the transverse view of the uterine cornu to each adnexa to bring the ovary into view. Raising and lowering the probe handle will move the beam through each ovary. If the ovary is imaged in the sagittal plane the handle is moved from medial to lateral (side to side). If bowel gas is obstructing the view gentle pressure is applied to bring the ovary into view.

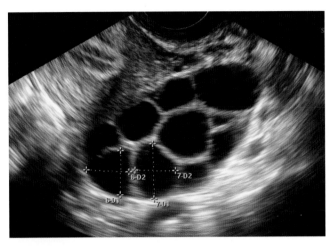

Figure 2.51 Left ovary seen lateral to the uterus.

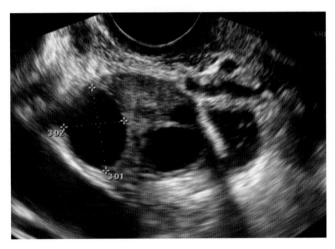

Figure 2.52 Right ovary seen medial to the iliac vessel.

At the completion of the examination the probe must be cleaned and disinfected using the Australasian Society for Ultrasound in Medicine (ASUM) protocols (www .asum.com.au) or as specified within the department guidelines.

ASUM Standards of Practice Statement

Ultrasound transducers are heat-sensitive items and as such will need to be disinfected using low-temperature chemical sterilis-ing/disinfecting agents or other approved automated systems.

Any products used for cleaning or disinfection must be compatible with the ultrasound equipment as determined by the ultrasound equipment manufacturer. The instructions for use for any ultrasound equipment must be consulted to ensure compatibility prior to using any type of disinfectant on their transducers. Care should be taken to follow each disinfectant manufacturer's labelled conditions for the use of their specific products. Directions for use are not interchangeable between formulations from either the same or different manufacturers.

J. Basseal and T. F. van de Mortel

Transabdominal Imaging

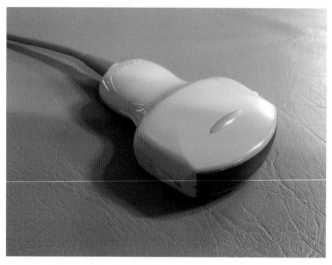

Figure 2.53 Transabdominal probe.

The transabdominal scan views the pelvic structures through the abdominal wall and a full bladder, enabling transmission of the beam without bowel gas obstructing the path. Filling the bladder elevates the anteverted uterus into a position perpendicular to the beam and provides a window to the lower pelvis, which allows the pelvic structures to be visualised and measured. In the sagittal plane the bladder can be assessed for optimal filling.

The curvilinear, lower frequency (2–5 MHz) probe allows for the pelvic organs, at depth, to be imaged. Using a lower frequency probe provides the depth; however, the resolution is not as clear as in TV imaging.

The probe is placed above the symphysis pubis and angled to obtain the best views of the uterus and ovaries. The ovaries can be seen posterior to the bladder wall and the beam can be angled through the bladder, in a diagonal direction to image the lateral aspects of the opposite side.

The uterus and ovaries are scanned in the longitudinal and transverse planes and measurements taken, the same as with the transvaginal approach. Adjust the depth, focus and the greyscale to optimise the images. The uterus is seen midline and the ovaries to the right and left lateral aspects of the uterus.

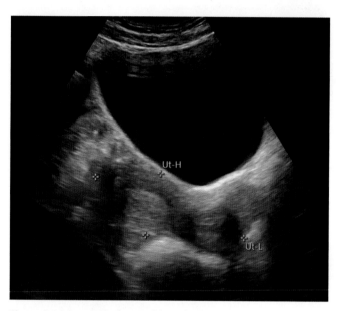

Figure 2.54 Longitudinal view of the pelvis.
Courtesy of E. Linton Kogarah Medical Imaging

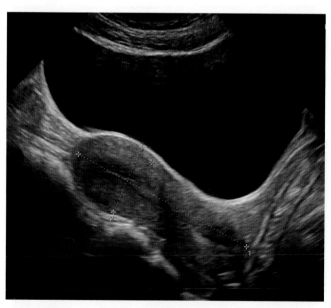

Figure 2.55 Transabdominal sagittal view of anteverted uterus. The full bladder anteriorly provides an acoustic window to image the uterus.
Courtesy of R. Gibson, Ultrasound Care

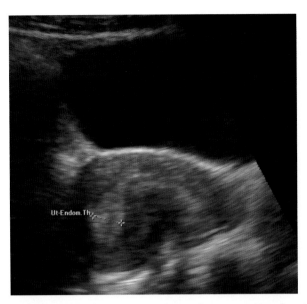

Figure 2.56 Transabdominal sagittal view of a retroverted/retroflexed uterus.

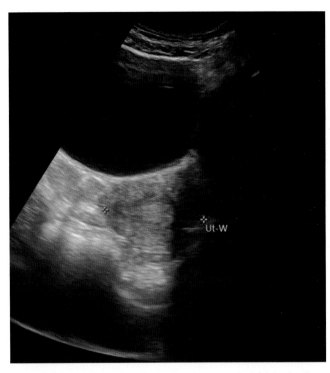

Figure 2.59 Transverse view of the uterus; however, the left lateral wall is shadowed by the refractive edge shadowing from the bladder anteriorly. To overcome this artifact, move the probe to the patient's right and angle towards the left.
Courtesy of E. Linton Kogarah Medical Imaging

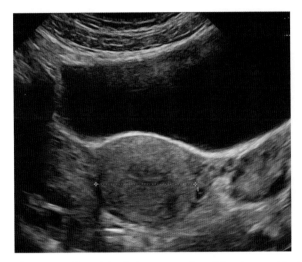

Figure 2.57 Transabdominal transverse view of the uterus and the left ovary.
Courtesy of R. Gibson, Ultrasound Care

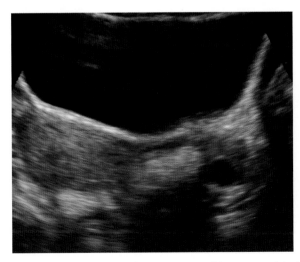

Figure 2.58 Transabdominal transverse view of the uterus and the left ovary. Bowel gas is seen between the structures and casting an acoustic shadow.

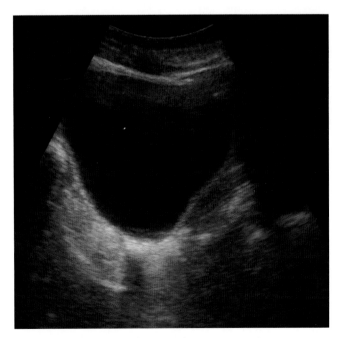

Figure 2.60 Transabdominal scan post hysterectomy.

A transabdominal scan may be required to demonstrate the full extent of a large fibroid due to the limited depth of the field of view with a transvaginal approach. Figures 2.61, 2.62

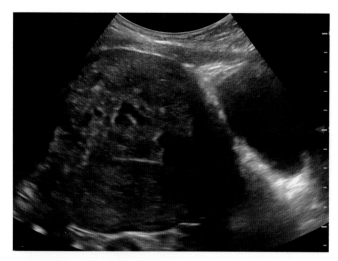

Figure 2.61 Large uterine fibroid uterus.

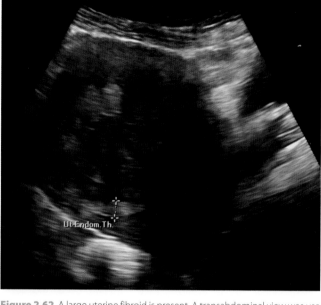

Figure 2.62 A large uterine fibroid is present. A transabdominal view was used to demonstrate the endometrium, which could not be seen transvaginally.

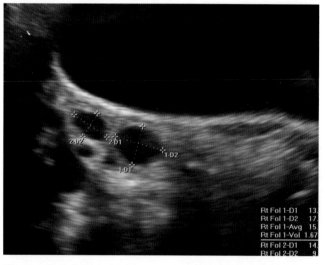

Figure 2.63 Follicles in the right ovary seen through the uterine bladder.

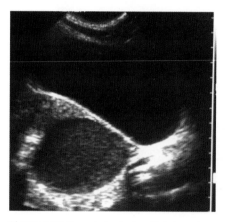

Figure 2.64 Transabdominal sagittal view of an endometrioma seen through the full urinary bladder.

(a)

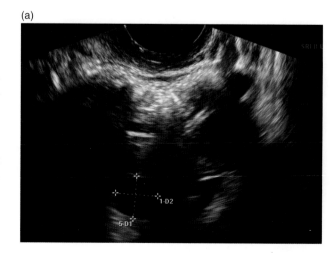

Ovaries located high in the abdomen and difficult to see or beyond the depth of penetration of the transvaginal beam may be found using the transabdominal view (Figure 2.66).

Place the probe in the transverse plane medial to the anterior iliac spine and slide inferiorly.

The transvaginal probe can be used if the TA probe is not available. A full bladder is not required, as the ovary is located close to the anterior wall and is within the field of view. (First, remove the used probe cover.) (Figures 2.65a and b)

(b)

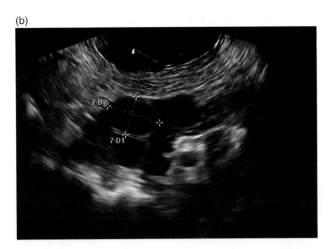

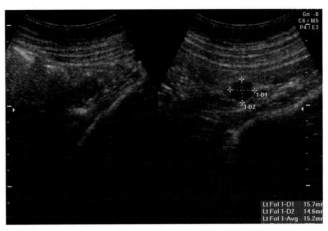

Figure 2.65 (a) The ovary is seen deep to the bowel, which is causing acoustic shadowing and giving a limited window to the ovary, located in the upper pelvic area. (b) The same patient as in (a). The ovary is located using a transabdominal approach with the TV probe.

Figure 2.66 The left ovary was located high in the pelvis, using the transabdominal probe, on a patient who had a uterine hysterectomy.

Chapter 3

Gynaecology Ultrasound

Transvaginal imaging of the pelvic area begins at the perineum. With the probe positioned at the opening of the vagina, in the sagittal plane, the image demonstrates the symphysis pubis anterior towards (left of image) and the rectum posterior (right of image).

As the probe is moved further into the vagina the cervix will come into view.

Once the cervix is seen, the probe is moved to observe the posterior wall of the cervix, to assess the position of the uterus in the pelvis. With small moves of the probe follow the line of the cervical canal into the body of the uterus.

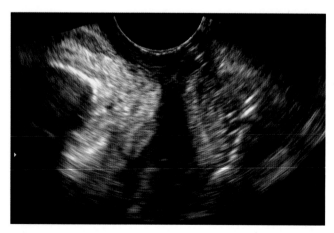

Figure 3.1 Begin with the probe in the sagittal plane – 12 o'clock.

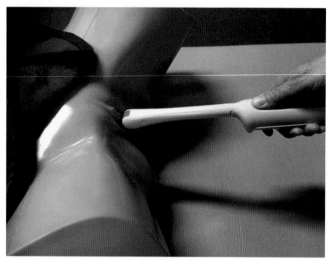

Figure 3.2 Transducer is on the peritoneum. The vagina is central, with the symphysis on the left seen as a bright echo with posterior acoustic shadowing and the rectum to the right of the hypoechoic vaginal echo.

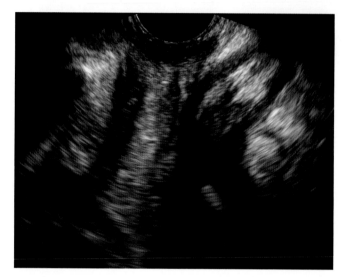

Figure 3.3 Hypoechoic bowel wall seen posterior to the vagina, to the right of the image.

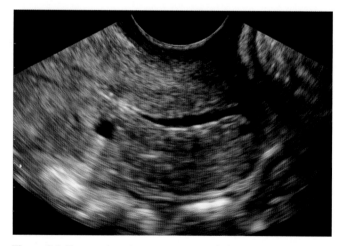

Figure 3.4 The transducer is now in contact with the cervix, with the cervical canal seen in the long axis view.

The Cervix

The cervix is located centrally in the pelvis supported by the cardinal ligament (the transverse cervical ligaments located laterally provide the major support to the cervix and uterus). Use the cervix as a reference point to assess the position of the uterus.

Under the effect of oestrogen in the late follicular phase, the endocervical canal contains mucus with a high fluid content.

Figures 3.5 to 3.8 show various positions of the uterine cervix in relation to the ultrasound probe. The posterior wall of the uterus is identified and can be followed to indicate the position of the fundus.

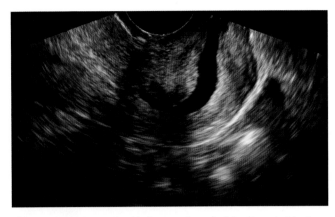

Figure 3.8 Uterine cervix with the posterior wall of the uterus in this view indicating the lie of the uterus in an anteverted position.

Anteverted Uterus

When the uterus is anteverted the fundus is seen towards the left side of the image. Move the probe to follow the cervical canal into the endometrial cavity, rotating the probe slightly, as required. Optimise the image by adjusting the depth, focus and gain and time gain compensation. (Figures 3.9 and 3.10)

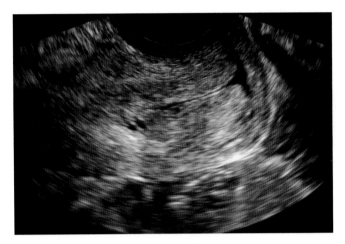

Figure 3.5 Uterine cervix in an anteverted uterus.

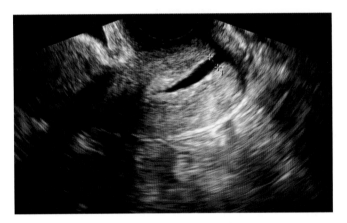

Figure 3.6 Mucus can be seen in the cervical canal.

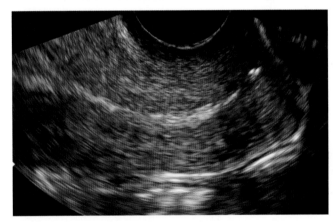

Figure 3.9 Cervix of an anteverted uterus.

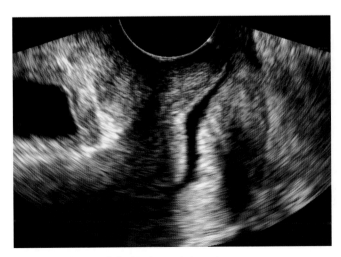

Figure 3.7 Cervix with fluid in the cervical canal.

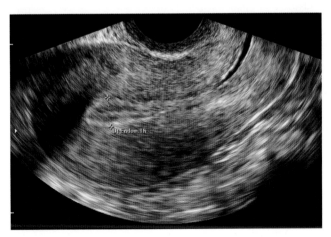

Figure 3.10 When the uterus is in an anteverted position the fundus is towards the left side of the image.

Retroverted Uterus

When the uterus is in a retroverted position, the fundus is located posterior to the cervix. Note the anterior and posterior walls of the cervix in Figure 3.11. While continuing to insert the probe, maintain contact with the cervix and follow the line of the cervical cavity into the body of the uterus. Raise the handle of the TV probe upwards and move the probe to the posterior fornix.

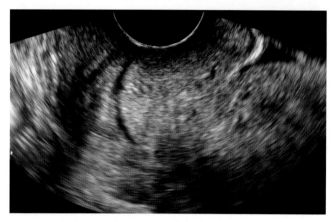

Figure 3.11 The cervix of a retroverted uterus.

As the probe is moved into the posterior fornix the endometrium can be positioned at 90 degrees to the beam. The uterine fundus will be seen on the right side of the monitor. (Figures 3.11 and 3.12)

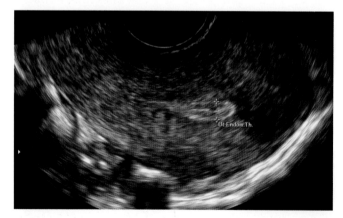

Figure 3.12 When the uterus is retroverted the fundus will be seen towards the right side of the image.

The Uterus in the Longitudinal Plane

When the uterus is in the mid position or longitudinal plane the endometrium appears more echogenic, due to the many reflections from the blood vessels and glands in the endometrium, being at 90 degrees to the beam. Beam width artifact is also seen at depth.

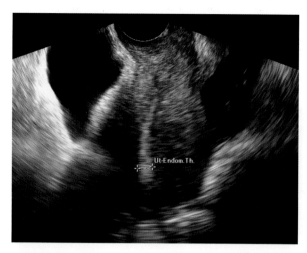

Figure 3.13 Uterus in the longitudinal plane and the tri-line appearance of the endometrium is difficult to demonstrate.

Scan the uterus completely in the sagittal plane from the right lateral margin through to the left side. Note the smooth outline, the texture of the myometrium, the presence of any pathology and its location and impact or distortion on the endometrium. If there is a Caesarean scar check its integrity.

Measurement of the Endometrium

Measure the endometrium in the mid, longitudinal plane, at the upper third, where it is usually the thickest. Callipers are placed on the outer edge of the basal layers, on the anterior and posterior aspects of the opposing endometrial layers, perpendicular to the cavity.

The thickness of the endometrium increases during the proliferative stage of the normal menstrual cycle. Post menses it is thin (<4 mm) and at ovulation may have increased to 12 mm.

The endometrial cavity is seen as an echogenic line through the uterus. The basal layer develops an echogenic appearance through the proliferative stage of the menstrual cycle, giving the tri-line appearance.

Callipers are placed across the full thickness of the endometrium from basal layer to the opposite basal layer and perpendicular to the uterine cavity.

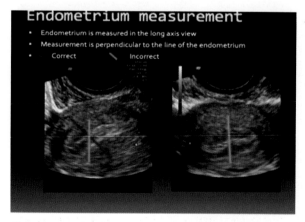

Figure 3.14 Endometrium is measured with the callipers perpendicular to the uterine cavity.

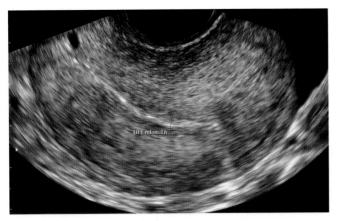

Figure 3.15 Retroverted uterus with thin endometrium (<2 mm).

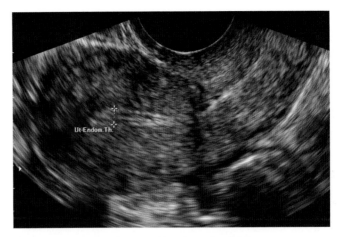

Figure 3.16 Anteverted uterus with endometrium 3.5 mm.

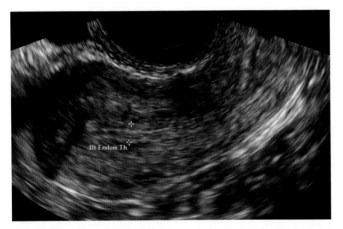

Figure 3.17 Endometrium measures 4.5 mm.

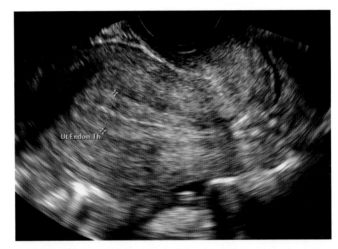

Figure 3.18 Endometrium measures 10 mm.

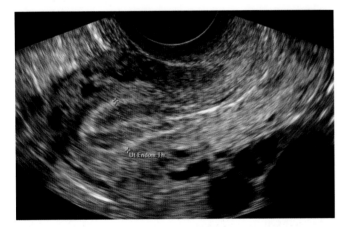

Figure 3.19 Anteverted uterus. Endometrium measures 12 mm.

Measurement of the Endometrium in a Retroverted Uterus

When the uterus is in a retroverted position, find the cervix first, ensure sufficient depth (field of view). Note the outline of the uterus coursing posteriorly or deep to the transducer position. Move the probe into the posterior fornix, by withdrawing it slightly, tilt the transducer towards the posterior aspect of the cervix and then gently push it deeper (Figures 3.20a and b).

(a)

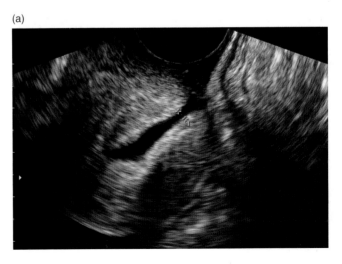

(b)

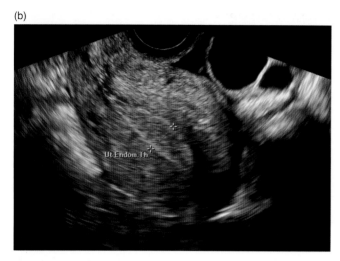

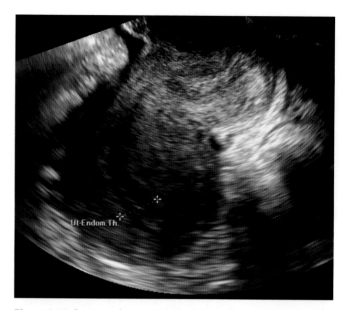

Figure 3.20 (a) The cervix is demonstrated and with gentle pressure move the probe deeper into the posterior fornix. (b) Retroverted uterus with probe in the posterior fornix.

Figure 3.23 Retroverted uterus with the probe in the anterior fornix.

The fundus of the uterus will be seen towards the right side of the screen.

Note: The posterior wall of the uterus is adjacent to the probe when the uterus is retroverted.

Measure the endometrium and check the uterus in the sagittal and transverse planes for any anomalies. (Figures 3.21 to 3.24)

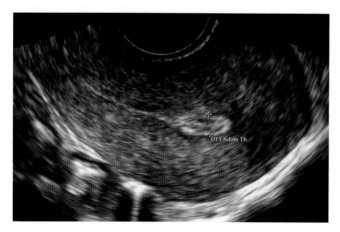

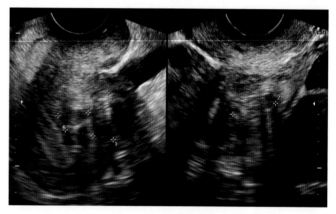

Figure 3.24 Bulky posterior uterine wall, caused by fibroids, seen in the long and transverse views, moves the endometrium in a more longitudinal plane.

Figure 3.21 Retroverted uterus – fundus towards the right side of the image.

Endometrium in the Longitudinal Plane

When the uterus is in an axial/longitudinal plane, the fundus is located deep to the probe and it can be difficult to get an optimal view of the endometrium (Figures 3.26a and b). This is due to the endometrium not being at 90 degrees to the transmitted beam and may give the appearance of a thickened endometrium, due to beam width artifact.

With this difficult scan, one option is to withdraw the probe to visualise the cervix and guide the probe into the posterior fornix; then manipulate the probe towards the uterine fundus and with a little more pressure, the uterus may rotate slightly, to get an appropriate view to measure.

It is nice to let the patient know you are having difficulty obtaining the appropriate image and to ask her to let you know if it is getting too uncomfortable. Often being in conversation relaxes the patient. (Figures 3.25, 3.26a,b, 3.27)

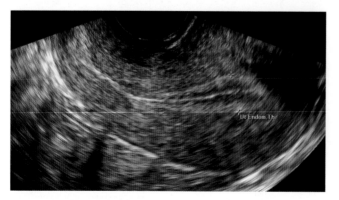

Figure 3.22 Retroverted uterus.

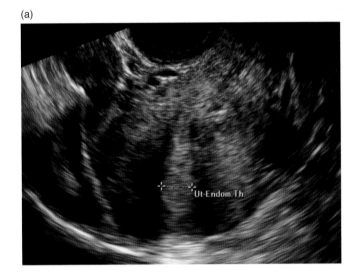

Figure 3.25 The endometrium in the axial plane appears echogenic and the margin is not well defined due to beam width artifact, making measurement difficult.

(a)

Figure 3.26 (a) Uterus in the axial plane. (b) With a little probe pressure curving the uterus and the endometrium can be seen with the tri-line appearance.

(b)

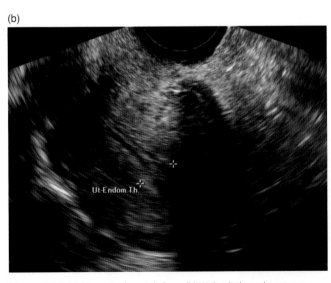

Suboptimal Images

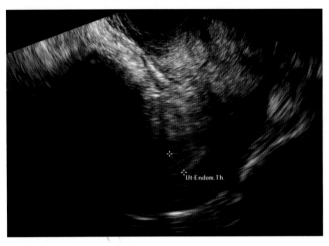

Figure 3.27 Long view of the uterus with gas in the bowel shadowing and obscuring the uterine fundus.

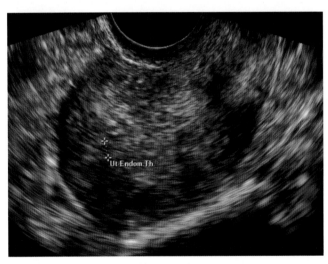

Figure 3.28 It is difficult to image the endometrium in a fibroid uterus.

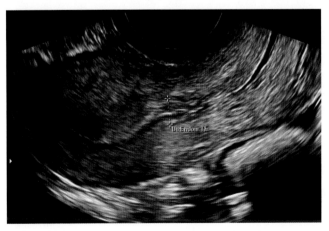

Figure 3.29 Due to adenomyosis in the anterior wall the endometrium is not clearly seen in the upper body of the uterus.

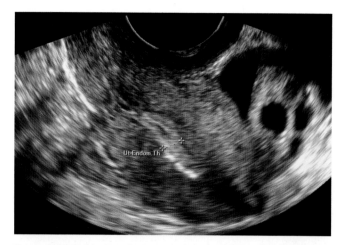

Figure 3.30 In this view of a retroverted uterus the endometrium is not fully visible and the measurement is of the anterior lining only (a little more probe pressure may move the uterus into a better view).

(a)

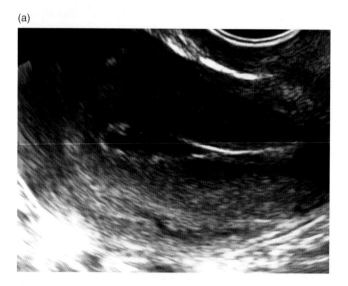

(b)

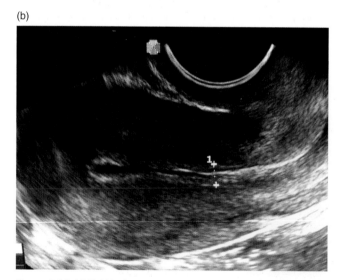

Figure 3.31 (a) Fluid in the uterine cavity must not be included in the endometrium measurement. (b) Manipulation of the probe enabled a section of the walls to appose and enable a single measurement or measure each side individually.

If the measurement is suboptimal, a repeat view at the end of the examination may provide a better window, for a more accurate measurement the endometrium. (Figures 3.28 to 3.32)

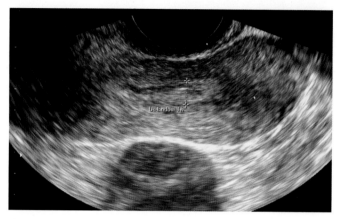

Figure 3.32 Transverse image of the uterus with distortion of the outline, between the transducer anteriorly and the spine posteriorly, by applying too much pressure with the probe.

Transverse View of the Uterus

From the longitudinal view of the endometrium, rotate the probe 90 degrees to image the uterus in the transverse plane. In this plane the right side of the patient is to the left of the screen and the left side of the patient will be to the right side of the screen. Scan from the cervix to the fundus (Figures 3.33a–e).

In the transverse plane the uterus is assessed for evidence of congenital variants, including arcuate uterus, subseptate, bicornuate uterus, unicornuate uterus and the presence of and the location of pathology. If pathology is present, images are taken in both longitudinal and transverse planes to demonstrate its location, size, echotexture and shape; if colour Doppler is available, the vasculature within or surrounding the lesion can be demonstrated.

3D ultrasound has the advantage to produce three-dimensional images which will demonstrate anomalies of the uterus and the uterine cavity.

(a)

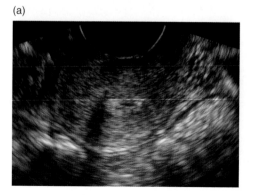

(b)

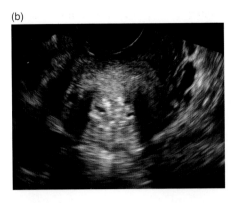

(c)

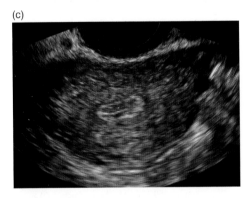

(d)

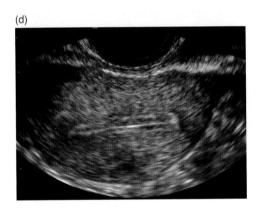

(e)

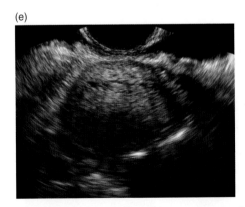

Figure 3.33 (a) Transverse view of the uterine cervix. (b) Isthmus of the uterus. (c) Transverse view of mid body of the uterus. The myometrium is hypoechoic compared to the surrounding tissues and the endometrial cavity shows the echogenic basal layer and the endometrial canal. (d) Transverse view of the fundal endometrium shows the wide upper section of the endometrial cavity. (e) Transverse view of the myometrium of the uterine fundus, above the endometrium.

When the uterus is in the long axis plane the beam will intersect the uterus in the coronal plane, with the fundus deep to the probe. The fundus can be imaged and assessed for any variation in the outline, as the probe is moved from the anterior to the posterior aspect.

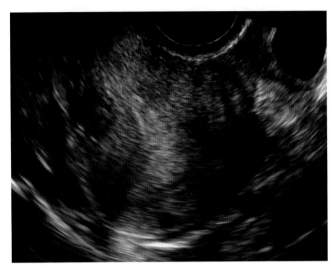

Figure 3.34 Coronal view of the endometrium.

The probe can be slightly rotated to follow the outer margin of the uterus and align the cornua symmetrically. (Figure 3.34)

Ultrasound of the Ovaries

The ovaries are usually located on the right and left lateral aspects of the uterus. They may, however, be posterior to the uterus or located above the fundus. Ensure sufficient depth to cover these areas.

To identify right and left ovaries move the probe from the transverse view of the uterus toward the left cornu and to the left adnexa. Locate the left ovary and then move the probe, still in the transverse plane to the right cornu and to the right adnexa. Locate the right ovary. Stimulated ovaries are more easily detected because of the presence of follicles.

During the follicular phase of the menstrual cycle a follicle (functional cyst) is seen as a fluid-filled structure on ultrasound imaging and should be round, thin walled and anechoic (no echoes) with posterior acoustic enhancement.

Primary and secondary follicles are microscopic in size and cannot be seen with ultrasound. Tertiary follicles have developed a fluid-filled sac called the antrum, which can be seen transvaginally, as 1–2 mm cystic spaces within the ovarian tissue. The presence of these in an unstimulated ovary will help to identify the tissue as the ovary and not the bowel or pelvic muscle.

Unstimulated ovaries are more difficult to see. They may appear as a slightly hypoechoic (darker) area, as seen in Figure 3.35. Optimise the image to demonstrate follicles 2 mm or less. The bowel will move with peristalsis, which can help to distinguish between ovary and bowel, when no follicles are present.

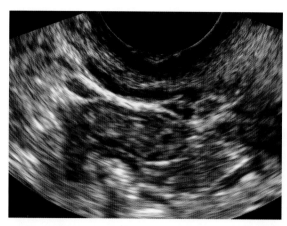

Figure 3.35 Unstimulated ovary, seen as slightly hypoechoic tissue with a 2 mm follicle.

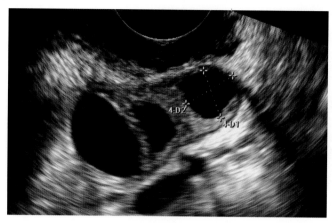

Figure 3.38 The left ovary outline is seen slightly hypoechoic to the surrounding pelvic tissues.

Graafian follicles are larger tertiary follicles, which have grown to a centimetre or more in diameter. In an unstimulated cycle several tertiary follicles grow to 8–10 mm on each ovary. One tertiary follicle will then accelerate in growth to become the dominant follicle, approximately 20 mm in diameter, and will release the mature secondary oocyte at ovulation. With ovarian stimulation more tertiary follicles grow to produce mature secondary oocytes (Sherwood, 2001, p. 738).

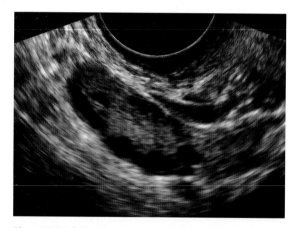

Figure 3.36 Right ovary located in the right adnexa. Tertiary follicles can be seen due to the fluid-filled space surrounding the oocyte.

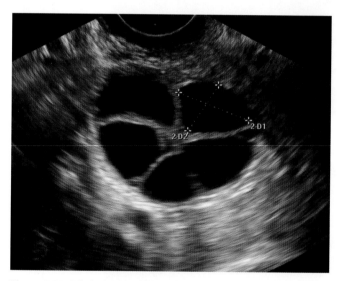

Figure 3.39 Follicle shape conforms to the space available. Follicle size is 17 mm.

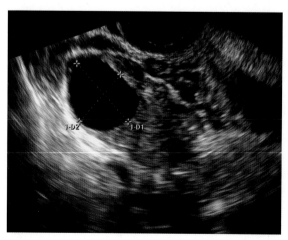

Figure 3.37 Dominant follicle is 21 mm.

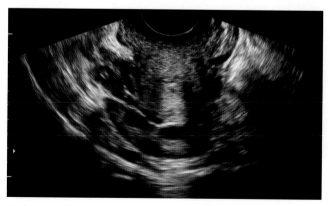

Figure 3.40 The ovary is located in the pouch of Douglas. Identify both ovaries first to confirm right and left.

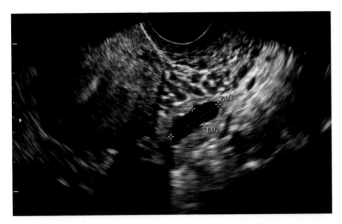

Figure 3.41 Blood vessels seen in the broad ligament, adjacent to the uterus at the top of the image. The left ovary is seen deep to the broad ligament and contains a follicle.

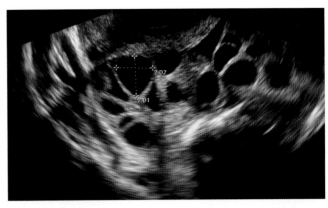

Figure 3.42 As the follicles enlarge, the ovaries can abut one another (kissing ovaries). Note the margins of the ovaries in real time before measurements are taken.

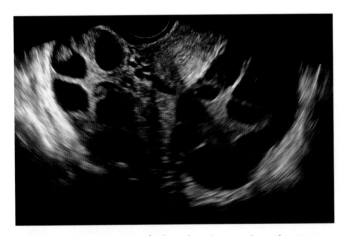

Figure 3.43 Transverse view of enlarged ovaries posterior to the uterus.

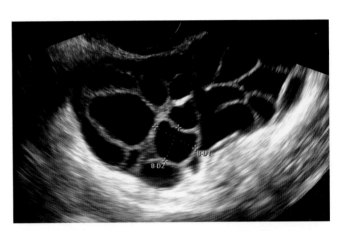

Figure 3.44 Enlarged ovaries abutting and located high in the pelvis. Time gain compensation could be reduced in the far field to reduce the brightness of the structures posterior to the ovaries in this image.

Follicle Measurements

Now that both ovaries have been identified, move the probe to visualise the entire ovary by raising and lowering the handle. The first sweep through the ovary will give an indication of the number of follicles present. On the return sweep, look at the sizes of the follicles to assess the number to be measured.

When there are multiple follicles, maintain the transducer in the same plane using the first follicle measured, as a reference point and continue measuring the follicles, systematically moving through the entire ovary. Count the total number of follicles and record measurements of follicles greater than 10 mm.

Measure each follicle in two planes at its widest diameter:

$$(L + H)/2 = \text{Mean diameter}$$

Move to the left ovary and measure the follicles in the same manner, as on the right. Record all data accurately at the conclusion of each examination.

When the ovary is located posterior to the uterus or above the fundus, use various approaches to optimise the best view. Abdominal pressure may move the ovary caudally. Rotate the probe to extend cephalad the "field of view" in the sagittal plane, if required. When the probe is in the sagittal plane the handle will be moved from side to side, to visualise the entire ovary.

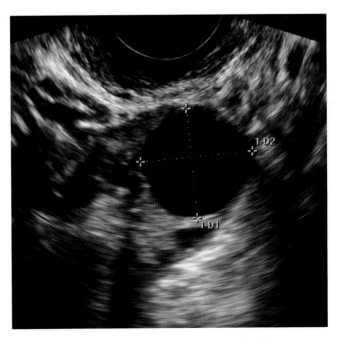

Figure 3.45 The dominant follicle is 21 mm in a natural cycle.

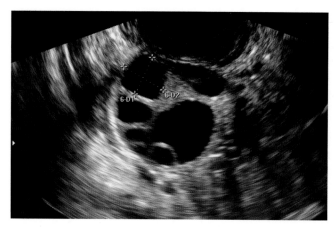

Figure 3.46 Right ovary located medial to the internal iliac vessels with follicles of various sizes.

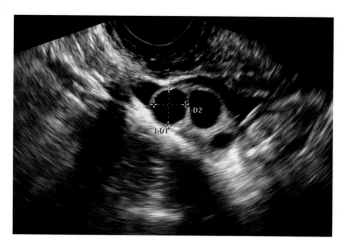

Figure 3.47 Free fluid in the peritoneal cavity adjacent to the ovary. Follicle size is 10 mm.

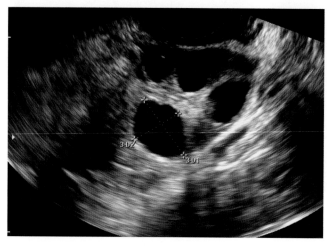

Figure 3.48 Left ovary located abutting the left lateral aspect of the uterus, medial to the pelvic wall. Follicle size is 14 mm.

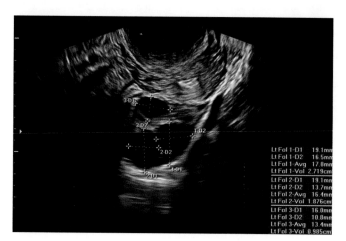

Lt Fol 1-D1	19.1mm
Lt Fol 1-D2	16.5mm
Lt Fol 1-Avg	17.8mm
Lt Fol 1-Vol	2.719cm
Lt Fol 2-D1	19.1mm
Lt Fol 2-D2	13.7mm
Lt Fol 2-Avg	16.4mm
Lt Fol 2-Vol	1.876cm
Lt Fol 3-D1	16.0mm
Lt Fol 3-D2	10.8mm
Lt Fol 3-Avg	13.4mm
Lt Fol 3-Vol	0.985cm

Figure 3.49 Multiple follicles can be measured in one view provided each is at the maximum diameter.

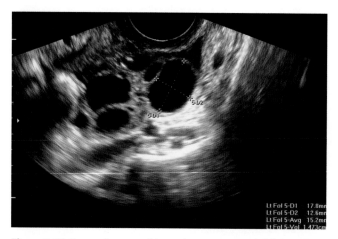

Lt Fol 5-D1	17.8mm
Lt Fol 5-D2	12.6mm
Lt Fol 5-Avg	15.2mm
Lt Fol 5-Vol	1.473cm

Figure 3.50 Use small moves of the probe to capture each follicle at the maximum diameter.

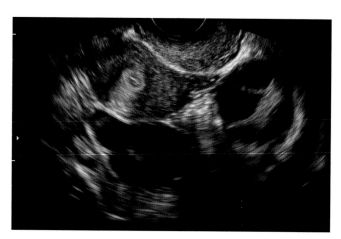

Figure 3.51 The right ovary is located deep to the uterus, which is leaning towards the right lateral pelvic wall.

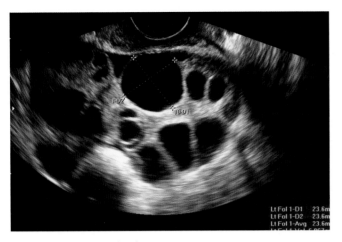

Figure 3.52 Hyperstimulated ovaries.

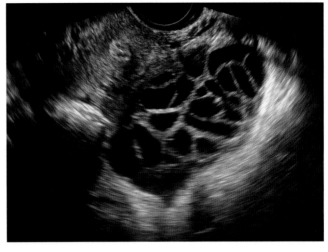

Figure 3.53 Polycystic ovary.

When the ovaries are polycystic it is important to measure the largest follicles. Count the total number of follicles by slowly scanning through the entire ovary, then scan again through the ovary from superior to inferior and establish the number and location of the largest follicles to measure, greater than 12 mm. Maintain the transducer in the same plane as you move through the ovary measuring each follicle.

Careful monitoring of these patients is required to prevent ovarian hyperstimulation syndrome.

Volume Measurement

When required, measurements for volume are recorded from two images taken at 90 degrees, long axis and cross-sectional axis. The structure of interest, that is, follicle, cyst, fibroid or other pathology is imaged at its maximum diameter in each view.

$$L \times W \times H \times 0.523 = \text{Volume}.$$

Uterine Pathology and Anomalies

The role of nurses conducting ultrasound in assisted conception cycle monitoring is to evaluate the endometrial thickness and document the size of each ovarian follicle present. Women should have undergone a formal diagnostic ultrasound prior to commencing a stimulation cycle; therefore any pathology present should have already been formally documented. However, if any pathology is identified on an assisted fertility cycle monitoring scan, it should be noted and brought to the attention of the treating doctor.

The following images demonstrate the most common anomalies seen in a gynaecology study.

Leiomyomas or Uterine Fibroid

Fibroids are benign tumours arising from the myometrium. Fibroids are extremely common, with one study of American women estimating a cumulative incidence of fibroids of 70–80% in women by the age of 50 years, with racial variation in frequency (Baird et al., 2003). Uterine sarcoma is a rare malignant tumour with an ultrasound appearance similar to that of fibroids. A meta-analysis of epidemiological studies estimated an overall incidence uterine sarcoma of 2.94 per 1,000 women undergoing surgery for a mass that preoperatively had been presumed to a benign fibroid. When stratified by age, the authors estimated a sarcoma incidence of less than 1 case per 500 women aged less than 30 years at the time of their surgery, compared to 10.1 cases per 1,000 women aged 75–79 years undergoing surgery (Brohl et al., 2015).

Fibroids may be submucosal (>50% of the fibroid is within the endometrial cavity), intramural (the majority of the fibroid is contained within the myometrium) or subserosal (>50% of the fibroid is located outside of the uterine myometrium). FIGO (International Federation of Gynaecology and Obstetrics) has provided a more detailed classification of fibroids, categorising from 0 to 8 depending of their location: 0, pedunculated within the cavity; 1, submucosal with <50% intramural; 2, submucosal with ≥50% of the fibroid intramural; 3, intramural with contact with the endometrium; 4, fibroid is completely intramural; 5, subserosal with ≥50% intramural; 6, subserosal with <50% intramural; 7, pedunculated subserosal; 8, other, for example, cervical (Munro et al., 2011).

Symptoms caused by fibroids are largely dependent on the location of the fibroid(s). Subserosal or cavity-distorting intramural fibroids may cause a number of problems including heavy menses and reduced fertility. A randomised controlled study reported that the removal of subserosal or submucosal-intramural fibroids resulted in an increased pregnancy rate (Casini et al., 2006). Guidelines produced on behalf of the American Society for Reproductive Medicine (Practice Committee of the American Society for Reproductive Medicine, 2017) state that there is insufficient evidence that any particular fibroid size, number or location (excluding submucosal and cavity distorting intramural fibroids) result in a reduced likelihood of pregnancy or an increased risk of miscarriage. Subserosal and non-cavity-distorting intramural fibroids are less likely to be symptomatic unless they grow to a large size and cause pressure related symptoms such as urinary frequency and abdominal enlargement or discomfort.

Fibroids may appear homogeneous or heterogeneous on ultrasound. Transabdominal sonography may be required to assess very large fibroids. The kidneys are checked for evidence of obstruction.

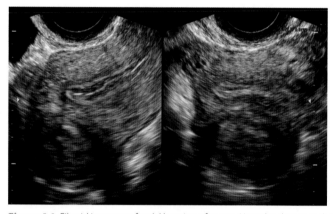

Figure 4.1 Fibroid in postero-fundal location of uterus. Note the change in the uterine outline.

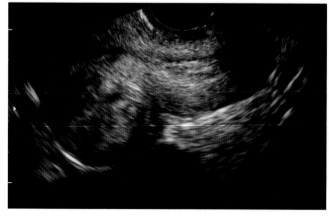

Figure 4.2 Subserous fibroid bulging outward causing the change in the uterine outline.

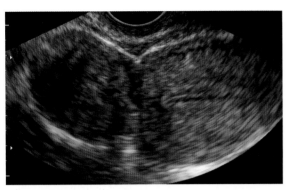

Figure 4.3 Sagittal view of the uterus with a subserous fibroid at the fundus. Note the distortion of the uterine outline.

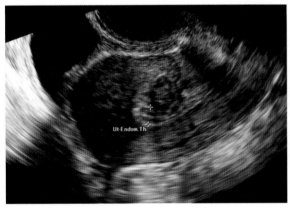

Figure 4.4 Submucous fibroid causing distortion of the endometrium.

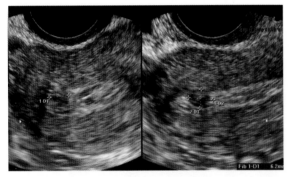

Figure 4.5 Submucous fibroid distorting the anterior endometrium.

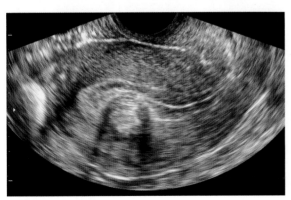

Figure 4.6 Submucous fibroid distorting the posterior endometrium.

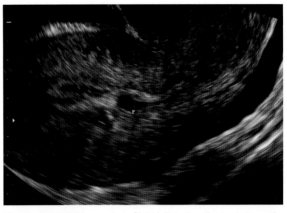

Figure 4.7 Small hypoechoic fibroid distorting the posterior endometrium. Free fluid noted in the pouch of Douglas.

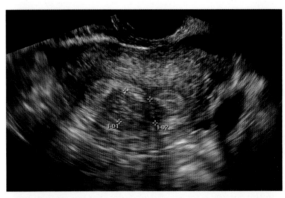

Figure 4.8 Transverse view, showing two small fibroids impacting on the posterior endometrium.

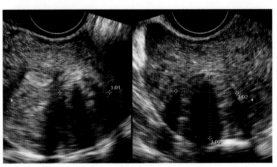

Figure 4.9 Dense fibrous tissue in the fibroid causes acoustic shadowing.

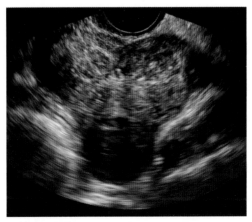

Figure 4.10 Multiple fibroids distorting the outline of the uterus and altering the texture of the myometrium.

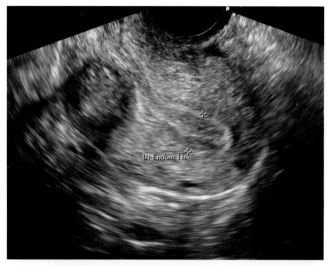

Figure 4.11 The dark (hypoechoic) area within the myometrium of the uterus indicates the pathology, a uterine fibroid.

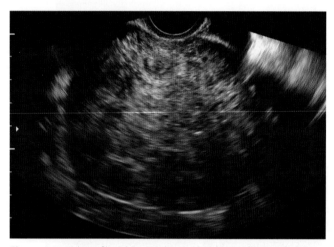

Figure 4.12 A large fibroid (12 cm diameter) makes it difficult to find the endometrium due to the mass effect on the body of the uterus.

Endometrial Polyp

Endometrial polys are localised overgrowths of endometrial glands and stroma, with a central vascular core, that project out from the lining of the endometrium. They are a relatively common incidental finding, with one study of 686 randomly selected Danish women aged 20–74 years reporting diagnosis of a polyp in 5.8% of premenopausal and 11.8% of postmenopausal women (Dreisler et al., 2009). The majority of polyps are benign, with one meta-analysis reporting 1.7% of polyps in premenopausal women were either hyperplastic or had focal malignant changes, with this proportion rising to 5.42% in postmenopausal women (Lee et al., 2010).

There is evidence that polyps may reduce pregnancy rates. Endometrial polyps may decrease fertility by physical mechanisms such as interference with implantation or sperm transport, or alterations in the immunological or cytokine microenvironment of the uterine cavity. A randomised controlled study of 215 infertile women with an endometrial polyp reported a statistically higher cumulative pregnancy rate of 51.4% after four intrauterine insemination cycles in women who underwent hysteroscopic polypectomy prior to fertility treatment compared to 25.4% in women who did not undergo polypectomy prior to their treatment ($p < 0.01$) (Perez-Medina et al., 2005).

The appearance of an endometrial polyp on ultrasound is an echogenic or isoechoic mass in the cavity of the uterus. Ultrasound diagnosis of endometrial polyps can be difficult, as the endometrial polyps can merge with the background echogenicity of the endometrium. Polyps should be imaged in both long and transverse planes to confirm.

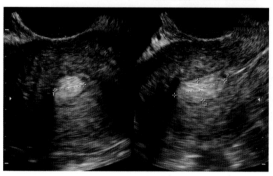

Figure 4.13 Uterine polyp within the endometrial cavity, seen as an echogenic structure.

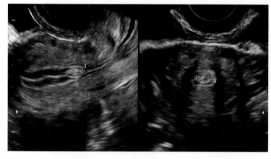

Figure 4.14 Longitudinal and transverse images of polyp.

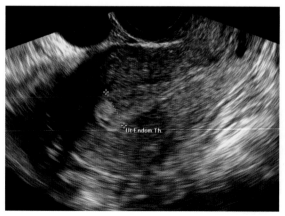

Figure 4.15 Endometrial polyp at the fundal endometrium.

(a)

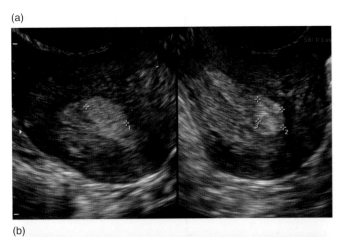

(b)

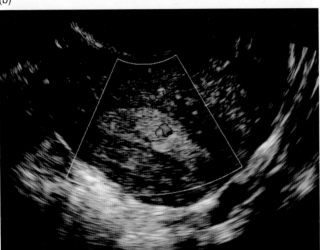

Figure 4.16 (a) Polyp seen as a slightly more echogenic mass within the endometrial cavity. (b) Blood vessel demonstrated in the polyp in Figure 4.16a.

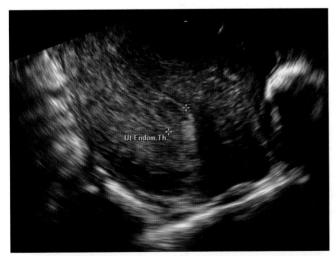

Figure 4.17 The echogenic area at the fundus of the endometrium in this retroverted uterus is not a polyp but accumulation of echoes from the curve of the basal layer and did not appear in the transverse view.

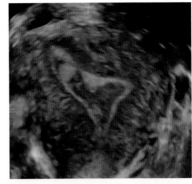

Figure 4.18 3D image of uterine cavity with polyps. Courtesy of E Linton Kogarah Medical Imaging

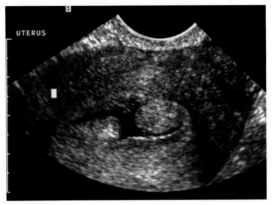

Figure 4.19 Sonohysterogram the infusion of saline showing two polyps outlined by the anechoic fluid.

(a)

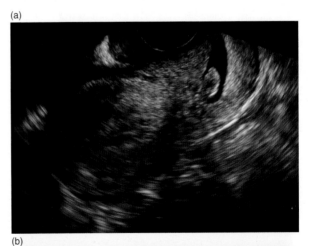

(b)

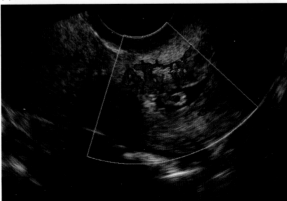

Figure 4.20 (a) Polyp seen in the cervical canal outlined by the cervical mucous which acts as a contrast agent. (b) Blood vessel to polyp seen in Figure 4.20b.

Cervical Stenosis

A significant amount of fluid in the uterine cavity requires careful evaluation. It may result from cervical stenosis. Benign causes include infection, polyps and submucous fibroids. Intrauterine fluid collections may also be associated with cervical or endometrial cancers. (Figure 4.21)

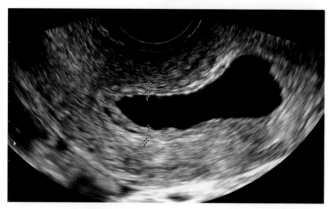

Figure 4.21 Fluid in the endometrial cavity, due to cervical stenosis.

Nabothian Cysts

Nabothian cysts or cervical cysts form when mucus-producing glands become clogged. They are a reasonably common incidental finding and measured only when above 10 mm. (Figures 4.22 and 4.23a,b)

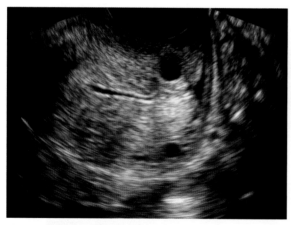

Figure 4.22 Nabothian cysts in cervix.

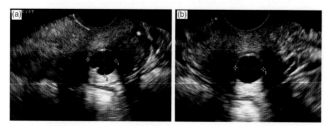

Figure 4.23 Nabothian cyst, 15 mm.

Cervical Fibroid

A cervical fibroid is a benign growth of fibrous tissue within the cervix. (Figure 4.24)

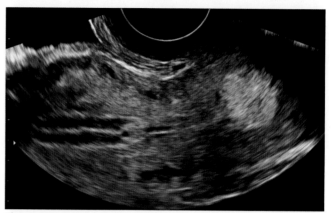

Figure 4.24 Longitudinal view of the uterus showing a dense mass in the cervix.

Cervical Suture

A cervical suture or cervical cerclage is a stitch in the cervix through the vagina to prevent early opening during pregnancy. (Figure 4.25a,b)

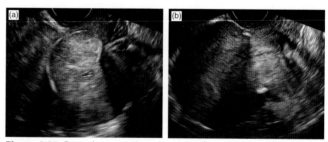

Figure 4.25 Cervical suture is the echogenic reflectors seen in transverse and longitudinal views of the cervix.

Subendometrial Uterine Layer

Figures 4.26–28 show variations from a 'normal' ultrasound appearance.

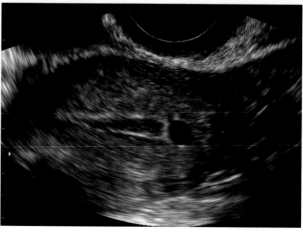

Figure 4.26 Cyst noted in the subendometrial layer.

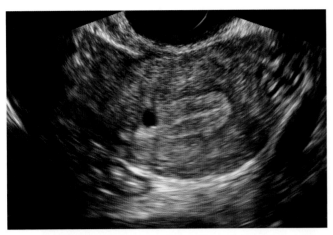

Figure 4.27 Cyst noted adjacent to the basal layer of the endometrium.

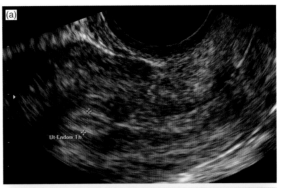

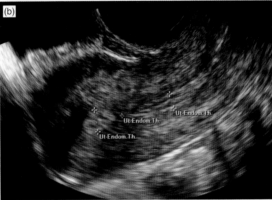

Figure 4.30 These images show the endometrium is not uniformly thickened (see measurements-5.5, 0.2, 3.7) and has an area showing no proliferation of endometrial tissue.

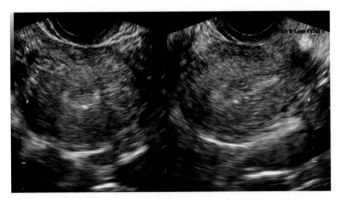

Figure 4.28 Echogenic foci, noted in the posterior basal layer.

Irregular Endometrium

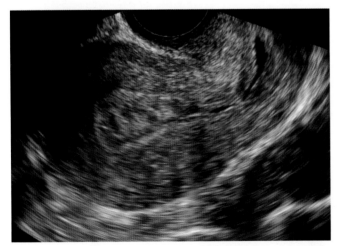

Figure 4.29 Normal endometrium; the irregular thickened appearance is not related to pathology.

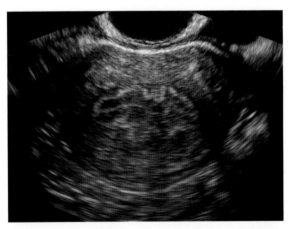

Figure 4.31 Transverse view of the endometrium. The basal layer of the endometrium has an irregular 'wavy' appearance.

Intrauterine adhesions require sonohysterography using saline to fill the cavity and provide contrast. Figures 4.30 and b show irregular thickening of the endometrium, and adhesions cannot be excluded.

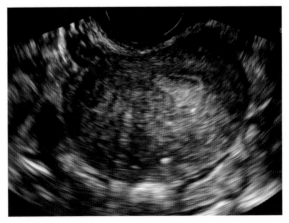

Figure 4.32 A bulky area of adenomyosis rotating the uterus and making the endometrium difficult to get an accurate AP measurement.

Congenital Uterine Anomalies

Embryologic development of the uterus is from two Müllerian ducts. Malformation occurs when there is failure of fusion, complete or partial, which results in a didelphic or bicornuate uterus. Failure of septum resorption to form a single uterine cavity results in a septate or subseptate uterus.

Complete failure of fusion results in uterus didelphys. More commonly, the cervix fuses and only the fundus fails to fuse, resulting in bicornuate uterus.

The arcuate uterus is the mildest fusion anomaly.

A septate or subseptate uterus results from failure of the median septum to resorb totally or partially.

A unicornuate uterus results if one Müllerian duct fails to develop. The degree of atresia varies.

Renal tract anomalies are often associated with uterine malformations.

Scanning through the uterus in the transverse plane, with the focus on the uterine fundus, will demonstrate congenital anomalies.

These examinations are often complex and 3D ultrasound is used to best demonstrate the anomalies. Jansen, R pp. 239–250

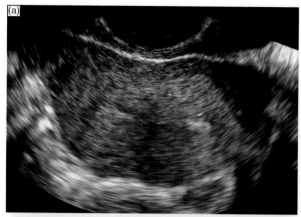

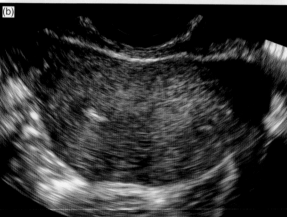

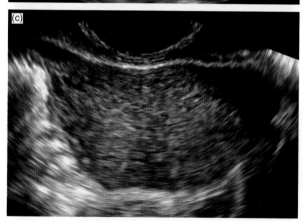

Figure 4.34 (a, b, c) The transverse sections through the fundal endometrium and the fundus of an arcuate uterus.

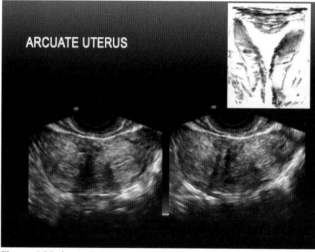

Figure 4.33 Arcuate uterus.

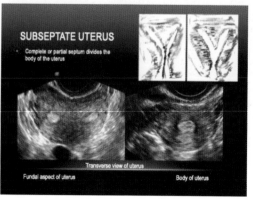

Figure 4.35 Septum is dividing the uterine cavity.

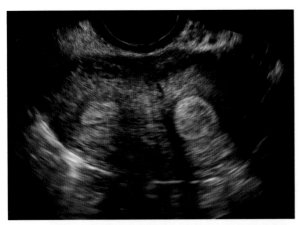

Figure 4.36 Subseptate uterus with asymmetrical thickness of the endometrium.

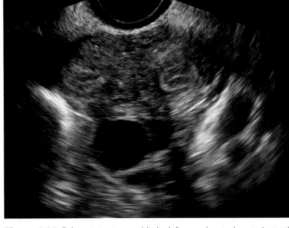

Figure 4.39 Subseptate uterus with the left ovary located posterior to the uterus.

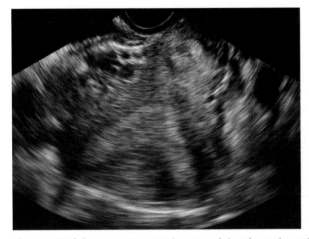

Figure 4.37 Subseptate uterus seen in a coronal view due to the position of the uterus in the longitudinal line of the pelvis.

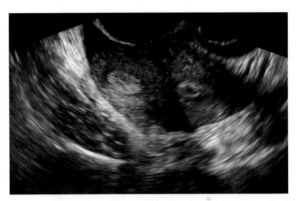

Figure 4.40 Transverse view of the uterine fundus showing asymmetrical thickening of the divided endometrium, in a subseptate uterus.

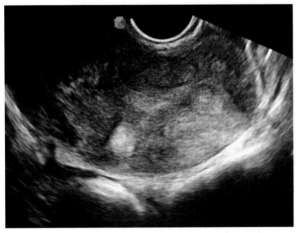

Figure 4.38 Coronal view of fundal endometrium in a subseptate uterus.

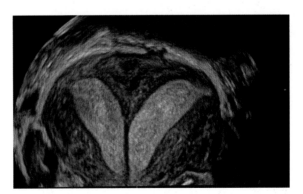

Figure 4.41 3D imaging demonstrates the septate uterus. Courtesy of R Gibson, Ultrasound Care

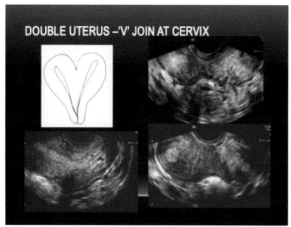

Figure 4.42 Bicornuate uterus.

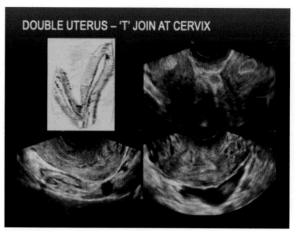

Figure 4.44 Didelphic uterus.

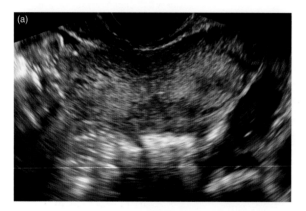

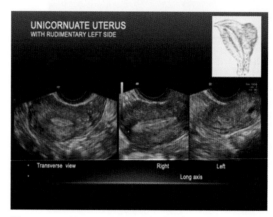

Figure 4.45 Unicornuate uterus with left rudimentary horn.

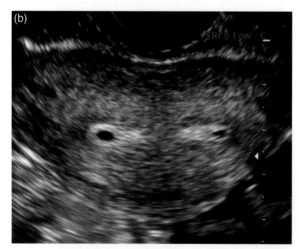

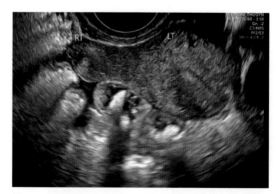

Figure 4.43 (a) Transverse view through the uterine fundus of a bicornuate uterus showing the appearance of two fundal outlines. (b) Transverse view through the divided endometrial cavity of the bicornuate uterus above.

Figure 4.46 Transverse view of the uterus showing a right rudimentary horn. Courtesy of R Gibson, Ultrasound Care

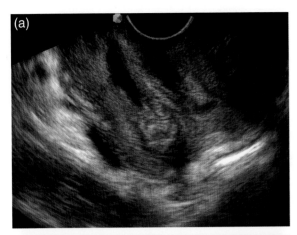

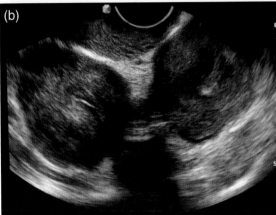

Figure 4.47 (a) Complete failure of fusion results in uterus didelphys, showing two cervical canals. (b) Complete failure of fusion results in uterus didelphys, showing two uterine bodies.

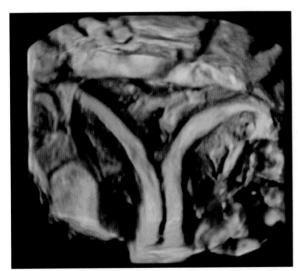

Figure 4.48 Septate uterus using 3D imaging. Courtesy of R Gibson, Ultrasound Care

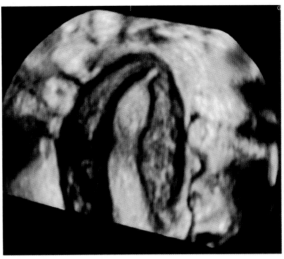

Figure 4.49 Unicornuate uterus. Courtesy of R Gibson, Ultrasound Care

Caesarean Scars

Caesarean scar defects can be identified using high-resolution transvaginal ultrasound. With the increase in cervical mucous in midcycle, acting as a contrast agent, the defects in the Caesarean scars are seen during the cycle monitoring ultrasound examinations:

- Deficient scars: detectable myometrial thinning
- Dehiscence: partial separation of the Caesarean scar
- Rupture: separation of the majority of a Caesarean scar
  Complications include
- Risk for subsequent pregnancies after primary Caesarean delivery
- Rupture or dehiscence at delivery
- Ectopic implantation
- Placenta accreta, increta, percreta
- Infertility (Naji O et al. 2012)

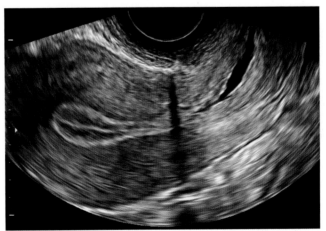

Figure 4.50 Caesarean scar indicated only by the acoustic shadow caused by the scar tissue.

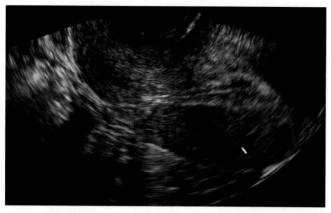

Figure 4.51 Retroverted uterus with Caesarean scar intact.

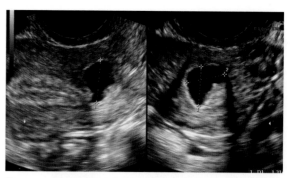

Figure 4.54 Cyst-like defect in the deep layer of the Caesarean scar.

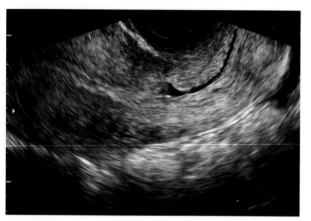

Figure 4.52 Defect in Caesarean scar; fluid provides contrast.

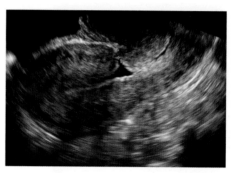

Figure 4.55 Small amount of fluid seen in the scar and in the body of the uterus. The myometrium measures 3 mm at the scar.

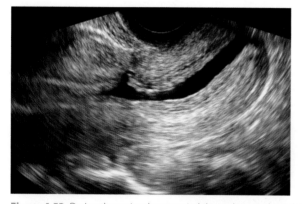

Figure 4.53 During the periovulatory period the endocervical canal contains mucus with a high fluid content, which provides excellent contrast.

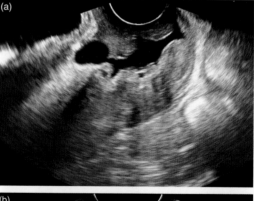

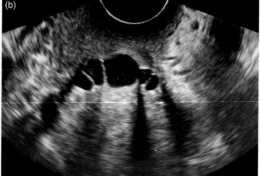

Figure 4.56 (a) Long axis view shows fluid in the cervical canal extends into the defect in the Caesarean scar. (b) Short axis view shows the Caesarean scar defect.

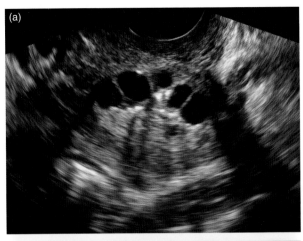

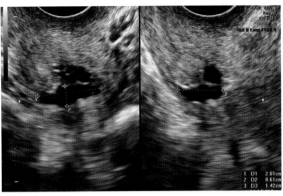

Figure 4.59 Images in transverse and long axis of scar in a retroverted uterus.

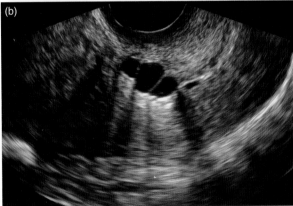

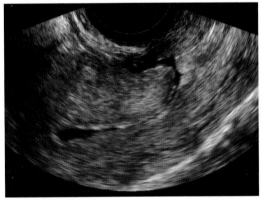

Figure 4.57 (a) Transverse view of the cystic pattern of the Caesarean scar. (b) Oblique/long view.

Figure 4.60 Careful manipulation of the probe in both longitudinal and transverse planes will demonstrate dehiscence of the scar and fluid in the endometrial cavity.

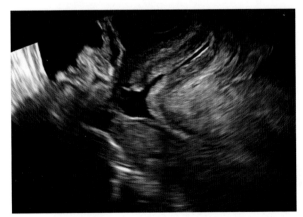

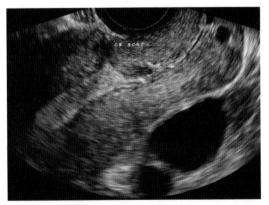

Figure 4.58 Dehiscence of the Caesarean scar in a retroverted uterus.

Figure 4.61 Caesarean scar seen in the lower uterine body distorting the endometrial cavity.

Endometriosis and Adenomyosis

Endometriosis

Endometriosis is a condition in which functional endometrial glands are located outside the uterine cavity. Common sites are the pelvic peritoneum, the ovaries, uterine ligaments and rectovaginal septum.

Abdominal pain coincides with menstruation as the glands respond to ovarian hormones, causing bleeding. Recurrent haemorrhage is followed by scarring and the formation of fibrous adhesions, distorting the ovaries and fallopian tubes, which may be a cause of infertility.

Small endometrial implants are too small to be imaged with vaginal sonography; however larger, localised endometriomas or 'chocolate cysts' can be detected with pelvic ultrasound.

Endometriomas on transvaginal scans appear as a unilocular or multilocular mass containing diffuse uniform echoes throughout (ground glass appearance), mildly thickened walls and acoustic enhancement. No vascularity is demonstrated inside the cyst using colour Doppler. A similar appearance may be seen with haemorrhagic cysts; however, these will resolve or decrease in size during the ensuing one or two menstrual cycles.

Endometriosis can infiltrate into the uterosacral ligaments, bowel, bladder and the vagina. Adhesions will cause the organs to be stuck together and the uterus and ovaries will not slide along the adjacent structures. This can be demonstrated by applying pressure on the uterus and ovaries and seeing the sliding movement of the structures against the adjacent tissues or alternately, by applying pressure on the abdomen above the symphysis pubis. These actions will elicit pain when pushing with the probe.

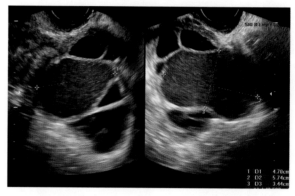

Figure 5.2 Endometriosis in the ovary with multiple follicles.

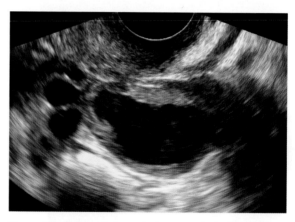

Figure 5.3 Endometriotic cyst in the ovary which is hypoechoic and has an irregular outline.

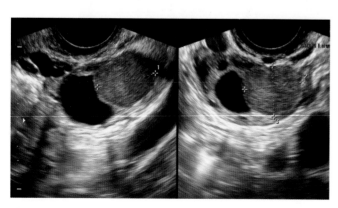

Figure 5.1 Endometrioma in the left ovary with follicle.

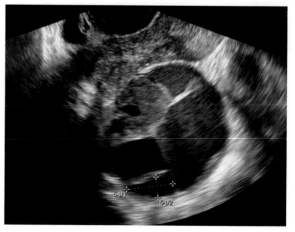

Figure 5.4 Multiple endometriotic cysts in the ovary.

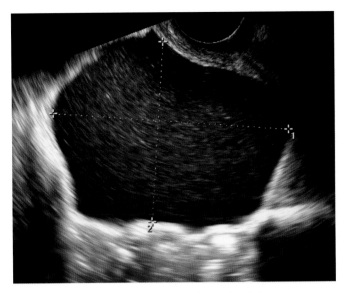

Figure 5.5 Large endometrioma seen as a hypoechoic lesion.

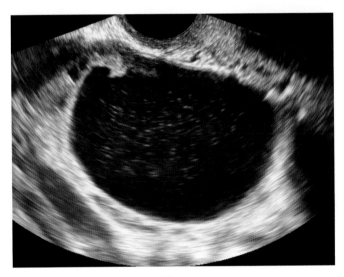

Figure 5.6 Endometrioma in the right ovary.

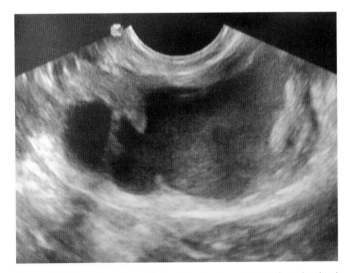

Figure 5.7 Extensive endometriosis with adhesions causing a large localised collection.

'Deep infiltrating endometriosis' (DIS) may be found in the bowel wall and the bladder with transvaginal scanning.

Deep infiltrating endometriosis (DIE) is seen as a hypoechoic mass lesion in the muscularis propria layer of the anterior bowel wall. It is found by following the bowel from the anal canal through the rectum. Detection of these lesions may be an incidental finding with sonography in a fertility clinic, and a referral for a comprehensive gynaecology ultrasound can expedite the referral to an endometriosis specialist who will work with a multidisciplinary team for treatment (Menakaya et al., 2015).

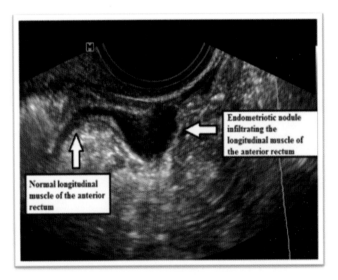

Figure 5.8 Endometrial nodule located in the rectal wall. Reproduced with permission from G Condos.

Infiltrating endometriosis into the bladder is seen as a hypoechoic mass extending through the wall of the bladder (Figures 5.9a–c).

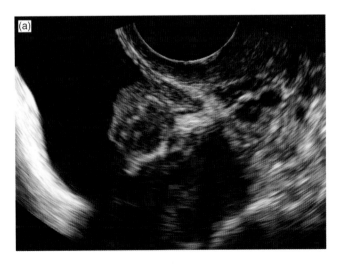

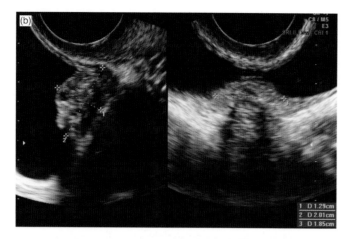

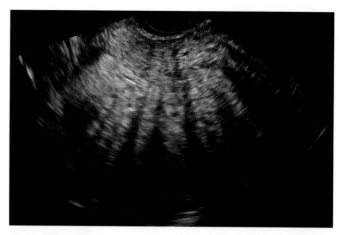

Figure 5.10 Adenomyosis partially obscuring the endometrium in the long axis view of the uterus.

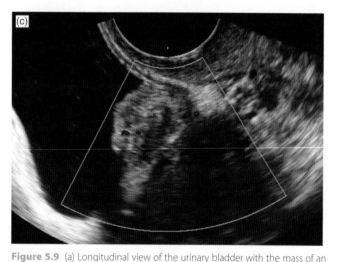

Figure 5.9 (a) Longitudinal view of the urinary bladder with the mass of an endometrial nodule extending into the cavity. (b) Long and transverse view of the endometrial nodule. (c) Longitudinal view with colour Doppler of the endometrial mass in the bladder.

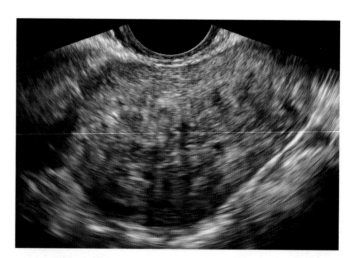

Figure 5.11 Adenomyosis demonstrating distortion of the smooth myometrial echogenicity.

Adenomyosis

Adenomyosis is a result of endometrial tissue within the myometrium. It may be localised or diffuse and cause a generalised or focal increase in the thickness of the myometrium. On transvaginal ultrasound, adenomyosis can produce uneven echoes from the myometrium. The ultrasound appearance may mimic leiomyomas; however, within the tissue, tiny cysts are present and there is no defined margin as seen with fibroids (Jansen, 2003, p. 234).

The change in the smooth texture of the uterine wall creates a 'fan effect' deep to the region of adenomyosis, in real-time imaging.

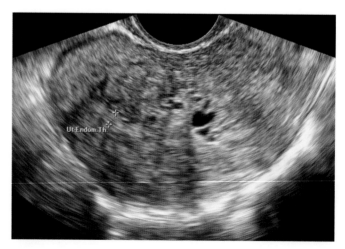

Figure 5.12 Cysts in the myometrium indicate adenomyosis.

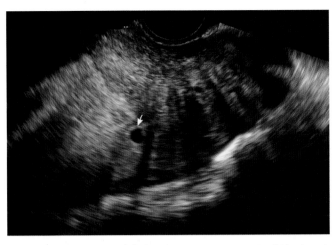

Figure 5.13 Localised area of adenomyosis causing extensive thickening of the myometrium.

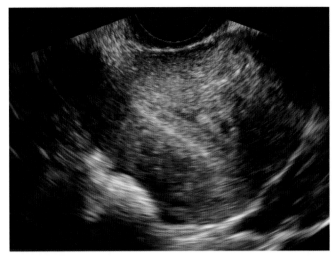

Figure 5.14 Adenomyosis seen as a thickening of the postero-fundal wall, in a retroverted uterus.

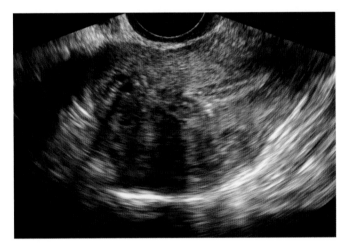

Figure 5.15 Adenomyosis.

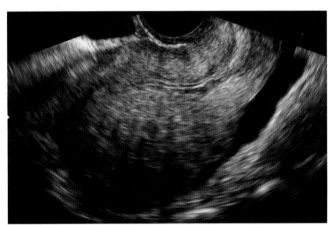

Figure 5.16 Adenomyosis of the posterior wall. Note the thickness of the myometrium in the affected area.

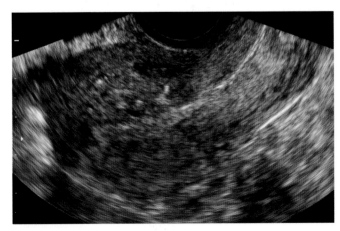

Figure 5.17 Tiny cysts in the area affected by adenomyosis can be seen in the anterior wall of the uterus.

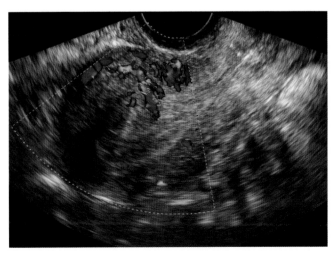

Figure 5.18 Increased blood vessels in the area of adenomyosis.

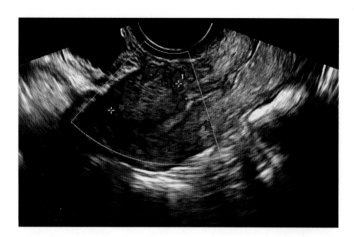

Figure 5.19 Increased blood vessels in the area of adenomyosis. Courtesy of J O'Brien, Genea

Ovarian Anomalies and Pathology

Chapter 6

Polycystic Ovaries

There are several different definitions of polycystic ovarian syndrome (PCOS). The most commonly used definition is the Rotterdam criteria, which states that the diagnosis of polycystic ovarian syndrome requires at least two of the following three criteria to be present: (1) oligo- or anovulation, (2) clinical and/or biochemical signs of hyperandrogenism, and (3) polycystic ovaries. The definition requires that all other possible causes of the aforementioned features must be excluded prior to the diagnosis of PCOS being made. Only one of the features required for the diagnosis of PCOS can be diagnosed on ultrasound, and other aetiologies for the required features cannot be excluded by ultrasound. Therefore it is not possible to diagnose a woman as having PCOS by ultrasound alone.

The number of follicles per ovary required to classify ovaries as being polycystic depends on the frequency of the ultrasound transducer being used. If the ultrasound transducer has a frequency of >8 MHz, then identification of 18 or more follicles per ovary is required before the ovaries can be considered polycystic; if the ultrasound transducer has a frequency of <8 MHz, 12 or more follicles per ovary must be identified to meet the criteria.

If a transabdominal approach is indicated (due to the patient being a virgo intacta or not tolerating a transvaginal ultrasound), only the ovarian volume should be reported; the threshold for polycystic ovaries is 10 mL or greater.

Diagnosis of PCOS in adolescent girls should not be based on ultrasound imaging of a high number of ovarian follicles, as there is a high incidence of healthy young women with multifollicular ovaries.

Unstimulated polycystic ovaries are seen with multiple small follicles located around the more dense ovarian stroma.

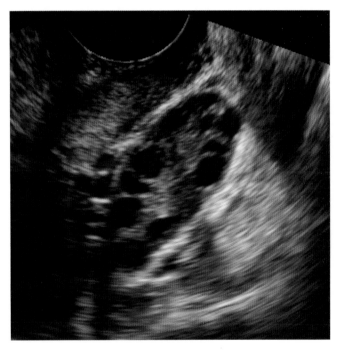

Figure 6.2 Polycystic ovary on day 8 of a stimulated cycle.

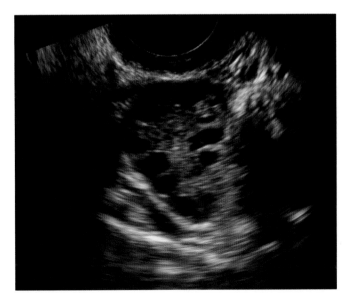

Figure 6.1 Polycystic ovary without stimulation.

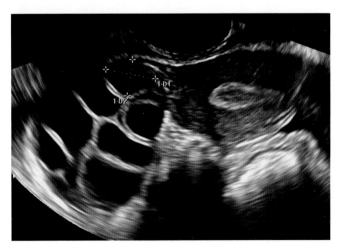

Figure 6.3 Polycystic right ovary lateral to the uterus.

(a)

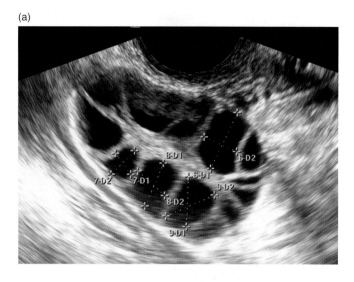

(b)

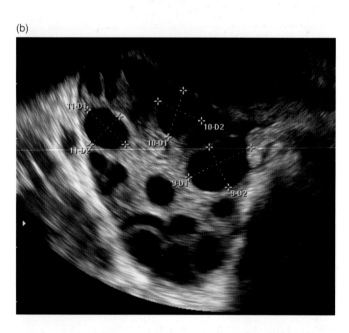

(c)

Figure 6.4 (a-c) Polycystic ovaries, with more than 12 follicles in one slice. (a) Multiple follicles. (b) Polycystic ovary. (c) Polycystic ovary.

(a)

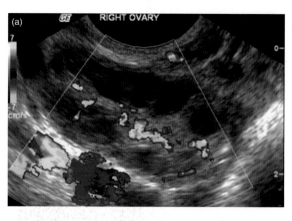

(b)

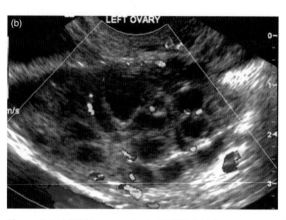

Figure 6.5 (a) Right ovary, patient with PCO. (b) Left ovary, same patient as in (a).

Ovarian Cyst

Cysts in the ovary most commonly are the result of 'mishaps' during the normal menstrual cycle resulting in follicular or corpus luteum cysts. They are less than 5 cm in diameter and may demonstrate thrombus in the lumen. They usually resolve spontaneously over the next one to two menstrual cycles (Callen, 1994). (Figures 6.6 and 6.7)

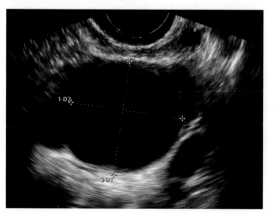

Figure 6.6 Thin-walled unilocular ovarian cyst.

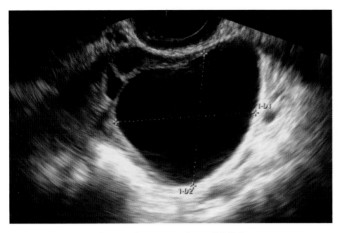

Figure 6.7 Retained cyst in the ovary with small follicles.

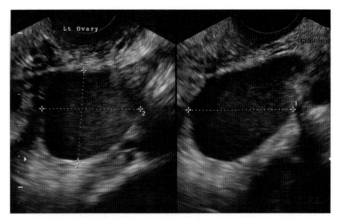

Figure 6.9 Haemorrhagic cyst.

When thin septa are seen within a cyst, the most common type of lesion, with this ultrasound appearance, is a serous cystadenoma. (Figure 6.8)

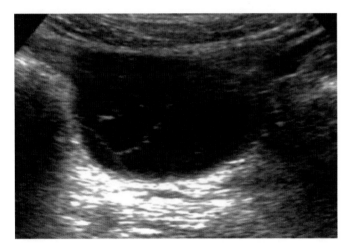

Figure 6.8 Loculated cyst contains thin septa.

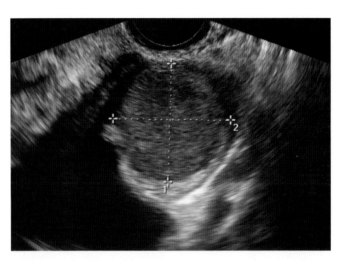

Figure 6.10 Haemorrhagic cysts contain low-level echoes.

Haemorrhagic Cysts

Haemorrhagic cyst is seen as a unilocular cystic mass measuring less than 5 cm with low-amplitude internal echoes within. The lesion can be monitored, by sonography, for resolution.

With colour Doppler, no flow is demonstrated within the interior of the mass. The appearances of a haemorrhagic cyst and an endometrioma appear similar on ultrasound. Clinical history and the day within the menstrual cycle are essential information. (Figures 6.9 to 6.19)

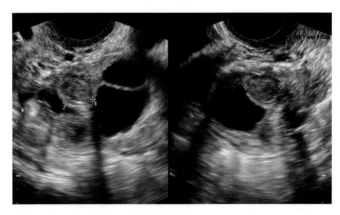

Figure 6.11 Small haemorrhagic ovarian cyst.

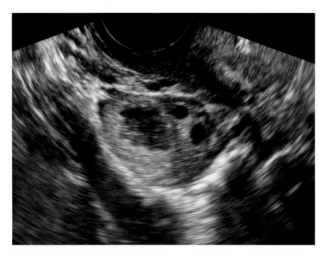

Figure 6.12 Corpus luteum and two small follicles seen in the right ovary.

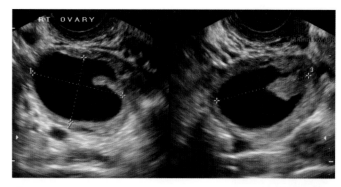

Figure 6.14 Complex ovarian cyst, seen as a cyst with a solid component on the side wall which may represent haemorrhage.

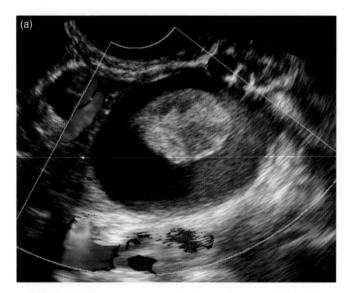

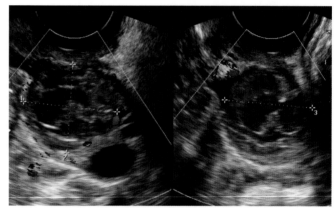

Figure 6.15 Haemorrhagic cyst (corpus luteum) showing no internal flow with colour Doppler.

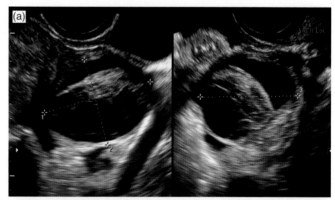

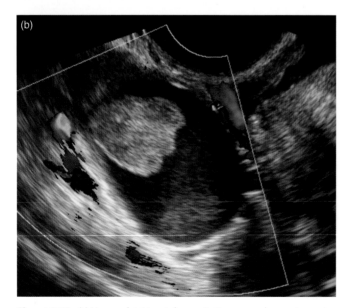

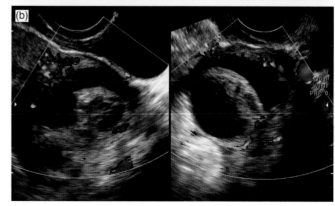

Figure 6.13 (a) Haemorrhagic cyst demonstrating a complex ovarian cyst appearance of cystic and solid components. Courtesy of J O'Brien, Genea (b) Long axis view of the haemorrhagic cyst.
Courtesy of J O'Brien, Genea

Figure 6.16 Haemorrhagic cyst. Colour Doppler shows that there is no vascularisation within the complex cyst.

Ovaries Post Egg Aspiration

Echoes are seen within the aspirated follicles. Bleeding into the peritoneal space around the ovary is seen in Fig.6.17 (Figures 6.17, 6.18, 6.19)

Cystic Teratoma (Dermoid Cyst)

Benign cystic teratoma or dermoid cysts are usually benign. They derive from a diversity of tissue such as hair, bone and sebaceous (oily) material, neural tissue and teeth which will produce a variety of ultrasound appearances including bright echoes, shadowing, fluid and a 'dermoid plug'. (Figures 6.20, 6.21, 6.22)

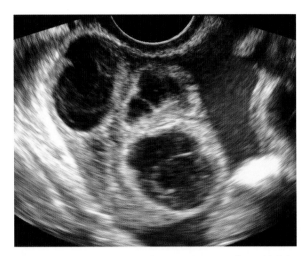

Figure 6.17 Ovary post egg collection, showing collapsed follicles. Small blood collection seen adjacent to the ovary.
Courtesy of J O'Brien, Genea

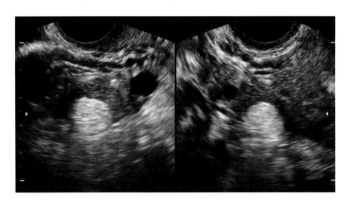

Figure 6.20 Dermoid cyst. Seen as an echogenic mass in the ovary.

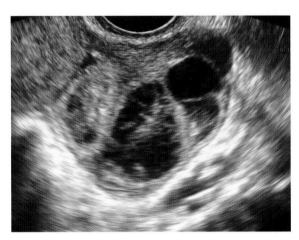

Figure 6.18 Collapsed follicles post aspiration.

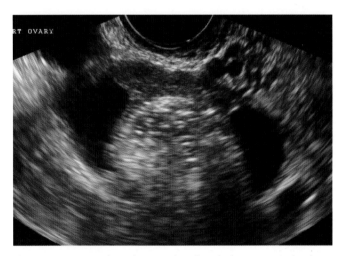

Figure 6.21 Dermoid cyst showing echoes from the hair content within the tumour.

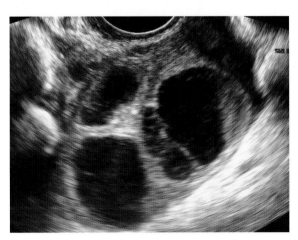

Figure 6.19 Ovary post aspiration.

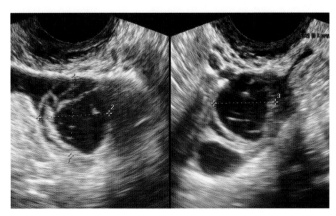

Figure 6.22 Dermoid cyst showing irregular echoes within.

Ovarian Malignancy

Cysts become suspicious of malignancy when there is an increase in the size, thickness of the septa, internal vascularisation and septal nodules are present. When a mass is found, describe the features in ultrasound terms: location, size, echogenicity, i.e. solid, cystic, complex and peripheral or internal vascularisation. Ultrasound provides an image, not a diagnosis.

(a)

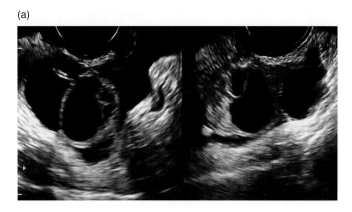

(b)

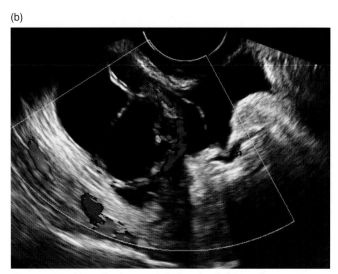

Figure 6.23   (a) Loculated cyst with thickened wall. (b) Vascularisation seen in the thickened wall of the loculated cyst raises the level of suspicion of malignancy. Courtesy of J O'Brien, Genea

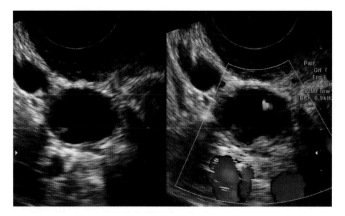

Figure 6.24   The addition of colour to the greyscale image shows vascularisation within the cyst.

Paraovarian Cyst

Paraovarian cysts are fluid filled cysts in the adnexa adjacent to the ovary and fallopian tube. They can be confused with ovarian follicles. Paraovarian cysts arise from remnants of the Wolffian duct in the mesosalpinx.

The margin of the ovary should be carefully followed to see if the cyst is within the ovary or outside.

The cyst can be separated from the ovary with pressure is applied by the transducer, when placed above and pushed between the two structures. (Figures 6.25a and 6.25b)

(a)

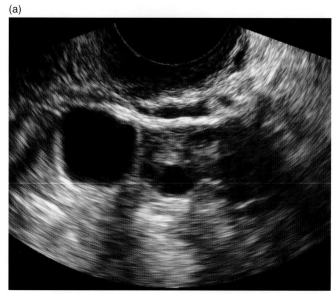

Figure 6.25   (a) No ovarian tissue encompassing cyst.

(b)

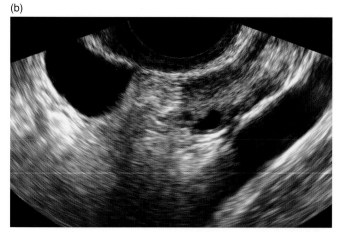

Figure 6.25   (b) Ovary and cyst separate with probe pressure.

Figures 6.26 and 6.27a and b were taken in 1980–81 using the Ausonics Octoson. Static images were obtained using the eight single-element transducers within a water bath to provide a wide field of view, demonstrating a panoramic view of the large cysts.

(a)

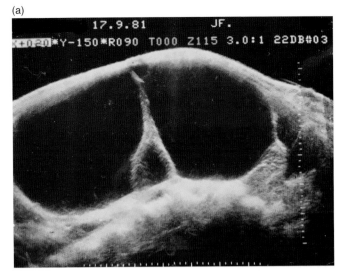

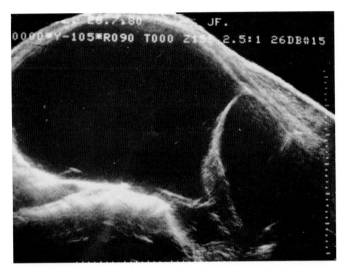

Figure 6.26 Huge unilocular paraovarian cyst seen in a midsagittal view.

(b)

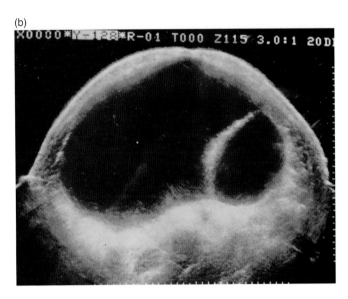

Figure 6.27 (a) Huge loculated paraovarian cyst seen in the midsagittal view. (b) Huge loculated paraovarian cyst. Transverse view of the image in Figure 6.27a.

Hydrosalpinx

Hydrosalpinx is a fluid accumulation in the fallopian tube which has become blocked, at the fimbrial end and the isthmus. This blockage can be caused by infection, sexually transmitted disease, previous sterilisation, endometriosis or surgery.

The ultrasound appearance of the fluid within the tube, can be confused with follicles; however, careful scanning and rotat-ing the probe will demonstrate the continuity of the fluid between one component to the next of the tortuous tube.

Corrugations in the wall of the distended tube may be seen. These corrugations are not obvious if the hydrosalpinx expan-sion of the tube has been longstanding.

(a)

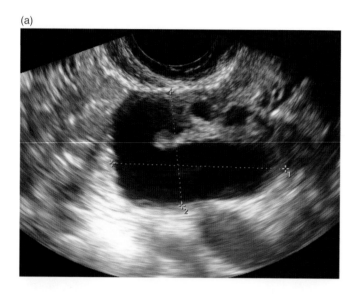

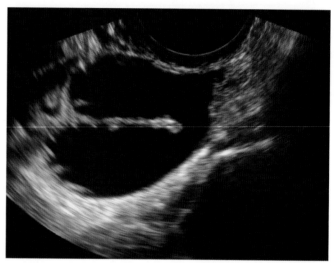

Figure 7.2 Hydrosalpinx. Note the continuity of fluid from one compartment to the next.

(b)

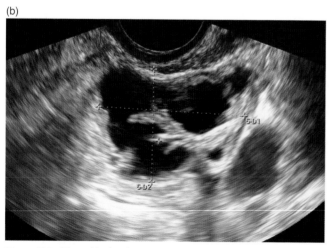

Figure 7.1 Bilateral hydrosalpinx is shown in (a) and (b). (a) Right adnexa. (b) Left adnexa.

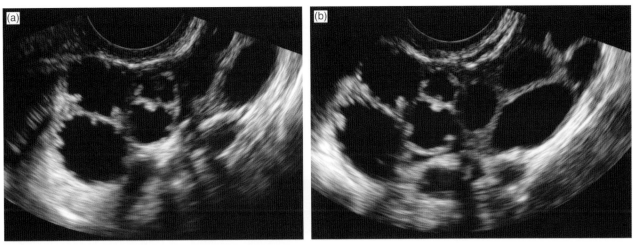

Figure 7.3 (a, b) Hydrosalpinx located adjacent to the left ovary. Note the corrugated lining of the fallopian tube and the smooth lining of the follicles in the ovary.

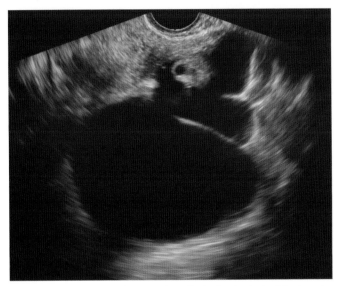

Figure 7.4 Hydrosalpinx showing a large fluid collection in the fallopian tube.

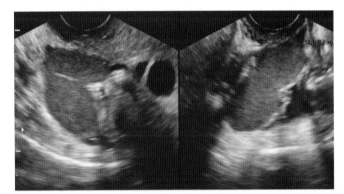

Figure 7.5 Fallopian tube distended with blood caused by a tubal ectopic pregnancy.

Ultrasound-Guided Procedures

Oocyte Retrieval

Transvaginal aspiration, guided by ultrasonography, is now a standard technique for oocyte retrieval.

The vaginal probe is covered in a sterile plastic sheath, with an attached needle guide. The guide is used to align with each follicle at its largest diameter. A 16–17-gauge needle is used to aspirate the fluid with the oocyte.

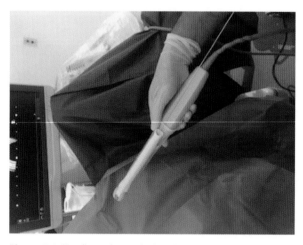

Figure 8.1 Needle guide attached to the TV probe.

Abdominal pressure can be used to stabilise the ovary or to move it to a more convenient location for aspiration.

Serious complications of oocyte retrieval are uncommon. Ultrasound provides visibility of the needle within the ovary and helps limit discomfort and ovarian trauma. (Figures 8.1, 8.2, 8.3)

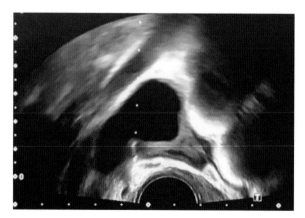

Figure 8.2 The image is inverted during the oocyte retrieval procedure. The needle tip can be positioned using the needle guide to align each follicle. Courtesy of R Gallagher, IVFAustralia

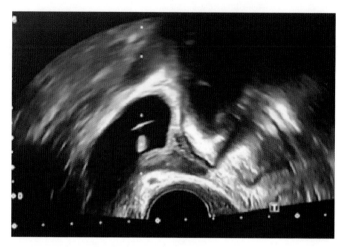

Figure 8.3 Needle tip can be seen within the follicle. Courtesy of R Gallagher, IVFAustralia

Embryo Transfer

Transabdominal scanning for catheter insertion into the uterus requires the beam to be focused on the cervix and lower uterine cavity. The bladder needs to be partially filled. The catheter is seen as an echogenic linear structure and the tip can be seen moving through the endometrial canal. Minor adjustments of the angle of the beam are required to maintain the image of the catheter.

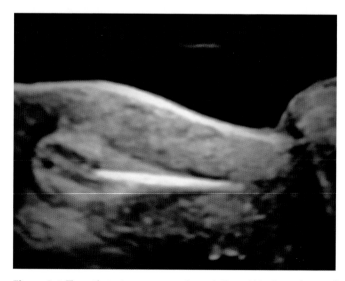

Figure 8.4 The catheter is seen as an echogenic line, within the endometrial cavity.

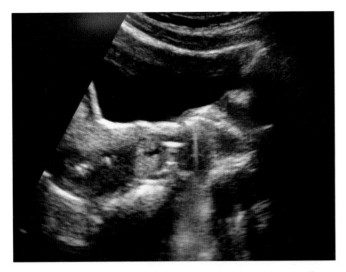

Figure 8.5 Transfer of the blastocyst using transabdominal scanning. The catheter can be followed during real-time imaging within the body of the uterus, seen here as echogenic dots within the body of the uterus.

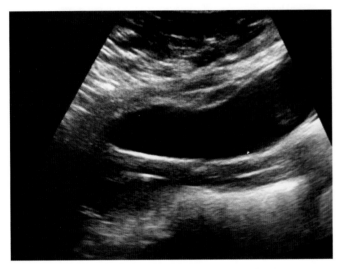

Figure 8.6 Transabdominal scan during the embryo transfer, demonstrates the echogenic catheter within the body of the uterus.

Using the transvaginal approach provides better resolution of the tip of the catheter as it is inserted into the body of the uterus.

A brief overview of the procedure is as follows. The patient is in a slight Trendelenburg position. A bivalve speculum is used to expose the cervix. The loaded catheter is inserted into the cervix and through the internal os. The speculum is removed and the transvaginal probe is inserted. The condom is wet with sterile normal saline.

The tip of the catheter is visualised and moved into position in the body of the uterus, under ultrasound guidance. Echoes are seen as the tiny amount of fluid, with the embryo, are injected into the cavity. (Figures 8.4, 8.5, 8.6)

Sonohysterography

In sonohysterography, saline is used to outline the uterine cavity. It is a procedure used to evaluate problems such as submucous fibroids, endometrial polyps, uterine adhesions and congenital uterine abnormalities. It is best to perform the procedure on day 5–10 of the menstrual cycle after the bleeding has stopped.

A bivalve speculum is used to expose the cervix. The catheter is inserted into the cervix and through the internal os. The speculum is removed and the transvaginal probe is inserted.

Normal saline fluid is injected. Ultrasound enables us see the fluid expand the cavity for evaluation of the lining of the uterus.

Figures 8.7a–e are a series of images to evaluate the polyp found with 2D imaging. Sonohysterography provides contrast around the polyp which can then be measured, localised and show the area of attachment to the uterine cavity.

(a)

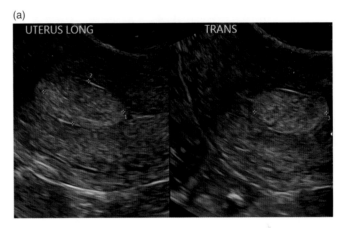

(b)

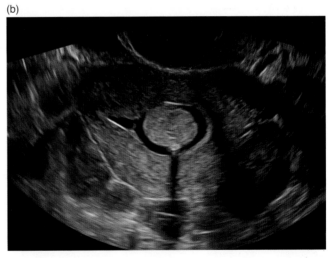

Figure 8.7 (a) 2D image of the polyp. Transverse view of the uterus. (b) The polyp is seen with the catheter posterior casting an acoustic shadow. Courtesy of E Linton Kogarah Medical Imaging

Sonohysterography with the addition of 3D imaging will produce high-quality images for referring clinicians.

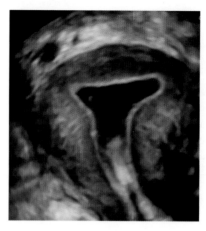

Figure 8.8 3D image of the uterus during sonohysterogram study, outlining the uterine cavity.
Courtesy of E Linton Kogarah Medical Imaging

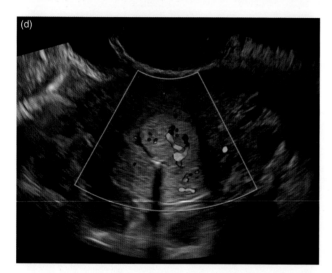

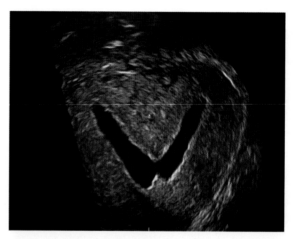

Figure 8.9 3D Sonohysterogram of subseptate uterus.
Courtesy of R Gibson, Ultrasound Care

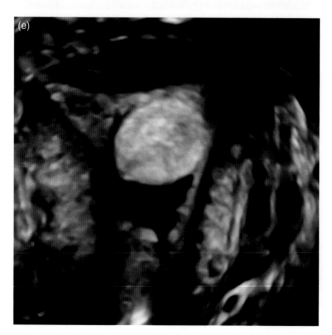

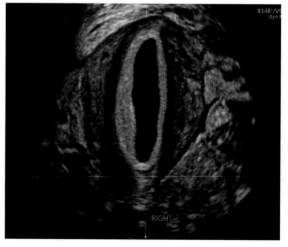

Figure 8.7 (c) Long axis view shows the polyp attached to the fundus of the uterus. The catheter can be seen. (d) Colour Doppler shows the feed vessel to the polyp. (e) 3D image of the polyp during sonohysterography.
Courtesy of E Linton Kogarah Medical Imaging

Figure 8.10 3D image of sonohysterogram of unicornuate uterus.
Courtesy of R Gibson, Ultrasound Care

Hysterosalpingo-contrast Sonography

Hysterosalpingo-contrast sonography (HyCoSy) requires the use of a contrast agent to visualise the patency of the fallopian tubes. The test is performed simply using an agitated saline–air mixture or a contrast agent called ExEm Foam.

A balloon catheter is used for this procedure to prevent the liquid leaking back through the cervix. The tiny balloon is slowly inflated with saline and can cause some discomfort. With the catheter remaining in the uterus the speculum is removed and the transvaginal probe inserted.

The initial part of the procedure is the sonohysterogram. Next, in order to see the fallopian tubes a small amount of contrast agent will be injected through the catheter. Tubal patency is confirmed when the contrast agent is seen flowing through each tube and spilling out around the ovaries.

These procedures, using contrast agents, can help define congenital abnormalities. The soft tissue and external contour of the uterus are seen with ultrasound, which is not demonstrated using X-ray hysterosalpingogram.

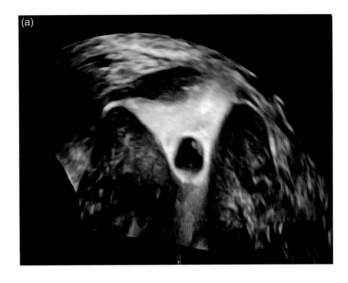

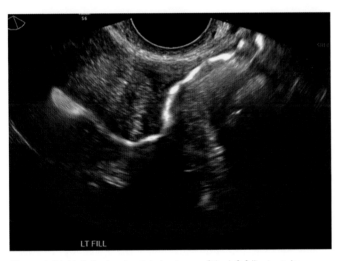

Figure 8.11 HyCoSy showing tubal patency of the left fallopian tube. Courtesy of R Gibson, Ultrasound Care

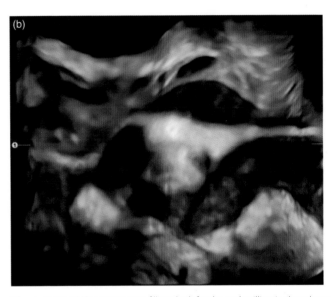

Figure 8.13 (a) Contrast is seen filling the left tube and spilling in the adnexa. (b) 3D image of HyCoSy showing contrast in both fallopian tubes. Courtesy of R Gibson, Ultrasound Care

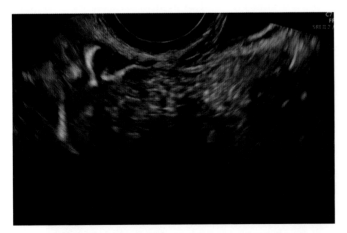

Figure 8.12 HyCoSy showing tubal patency of the right fallopian tube. Courtesy of R Gibson, Ultrasound Care

First Trimester Pregnancy

Sonography of first trimester pregnancy will determine the location of the gestational sac, viability, gestational age and assessment of multifetal pregnancy.

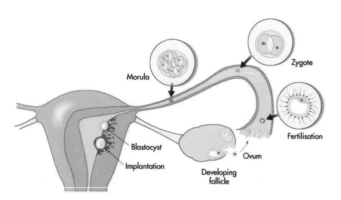

Figure 9.1 Normal fertilisation and implantation.

Elevated β-hCG in the maternal serum or urine is an indication of pregnancy. Once the hCG levels reach 1,000–2,000 mIU/ml a transvaginal ultrasound should be able to demonstrate a gestational sac.

At 5 weeks an intrauterine gestation sac is seen as an echogenic ring within the decidual lining of the uterine cavity.

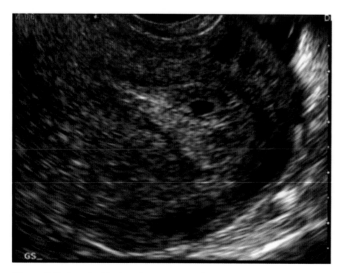

Figure 9.2 Intradecidual sac in a retroverted uterus.

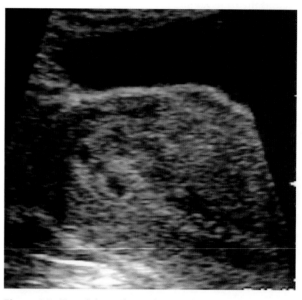

Figure 9.3 Transabdominal scan showing the double 'ring sign' of the decidua with the echogenic trophoblastic, implantation ring surrounding the gestational sac.

The yolk sac is normally the first structure seen within the gestation sac and is connected to the fetus by the vitaline duct. It can be seen transvaginally when the mean sac diameter (MSD) is 8 mm and transabdominally when the MSD measures 20 mm. It is a round anechoic structure and should not be calcified or misshapen. Measurement are from inner to inner diameter and should be less than 6 mm.

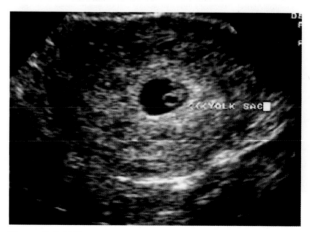

Figure 9.4 Yolk sac.

After 6 weeks the fetal pole and cardiac activity can be seen. Once the fetal pole is visualised the crown–rump Length (CRL) is the most accurate measurement for dating the pregnancy. A well-performed CRL in the first trimester is accurate to 5–7 days.

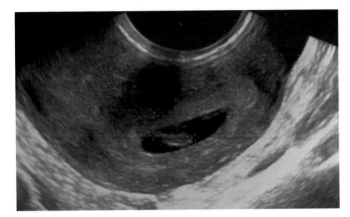

Figure 9.5 CRL measurement of the fetal pole 6w5d.

Charts are available from 6 weeks 3 days when the CRL is 5 mm. Do not include the yolk sac in the CRL measurement. The CRL measurements are used until 12 weeks when the fetus begins to curl into the fetal position.

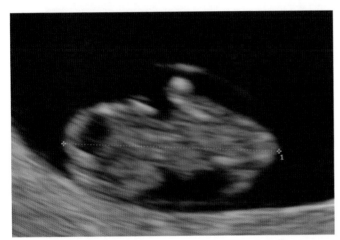

Figure 9.6 CRL measurement of 8-week fetus.

Transvaginal scanning will enable early pregnancy features to be seen earlier than with transabdominal scanning. Table 9.1 shows the detection of embryonic landmarks using transvaginal and transabdominal ultrasound. The gestational sac is surrounded by the echogenic trophoblastic ring within the decidua.

Table 9.1 Ultrasound findings in early pregnancy

Finding	Transvaginal	Transabdominal
Gest. Sac	4.5 weeks	5 weeks
Yolk Sac	5 weeks	5.5 weeks
Fetal pole	5.5 weeks	6 weeks
FHM	6 weeks	6.5 weeks

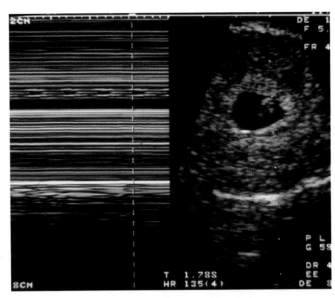

Figure 9.7 Fetal heart movement recorded (FHM 135) using M-mode.

The presence of a corpus luteum in the ovary should also be noted.

- FHM – detected from 6th week
- M-mode = motion mode
- M-mode is a measure of distance over time
- Single dimension time display that represents the motion of various reflectors

The amnion forms around the fetus within the chorionic sac. With the production of fetal urine, the amnion will expand rapidly after 9 weeks and adhere to the outer chorion by 14 weeks' gestation.

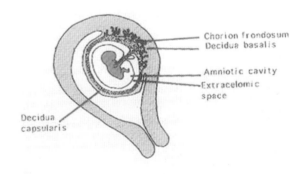

Figure 9.8 Development of the placenta and the amnion surrounding the fetus.

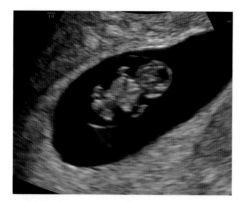

Figure 9.9 The 8-week fetus is within the amniotic cavity and the head, body and limb buds can be distinguished.
Courtesy of R Gibson, Ultrasound Care

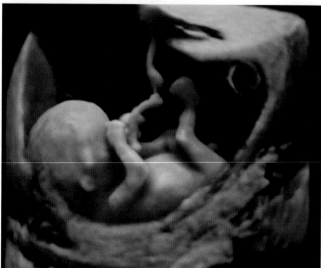

Figure 9.10 3D image of fetus at 10w5d.
Courtesy of R Gibson, Ultrasound Care

Multiple Pregnancy

Multiple pregnancy occurs when to two or more fetuses develop simultaneously in the womb. Twin pregnancy occurs when one fertilised zygote splits into two (monozygotic or identical twins) or two eggs are fertilised by separate sperm (dizygotic or fraternal twins).

Dizygotic twins = dichorionic–diamniotic twins

Implantation of monozygotic pregnancy varies, depending on the time of division.

1–4 days (morula) = dichorionic–diamniotic twins

4–8 days (blastocyst) = monochorionic–diamniotic twins

1–2 weeks = monochorionic–monoamniotic twins

>2 weeks = conjoined twins

Chorionicity is best assessed in early pregnancy with the chorionic ring surrounding each fetus (dichorionic) or two embryos in a single sac (monochorionic).

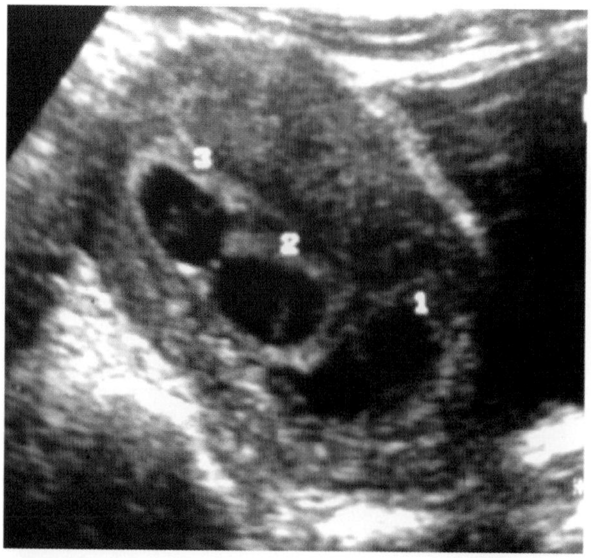

Figure 9.11 Triplet pregnancy, showing separate chorionic rings around each sac.

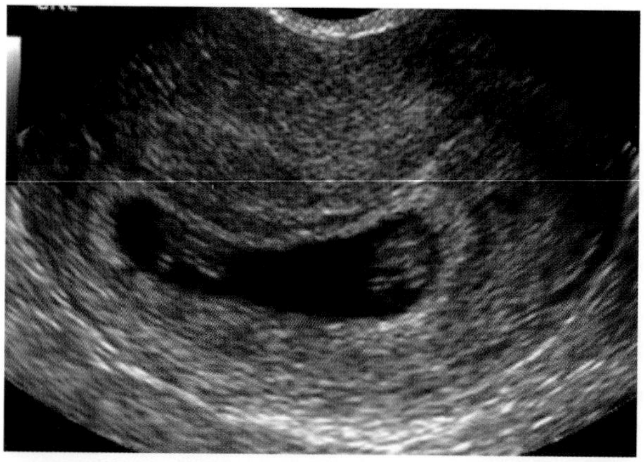

Figure 9.12 Monochorionic twin pregnancy showing two embryos in one chorionic sac.

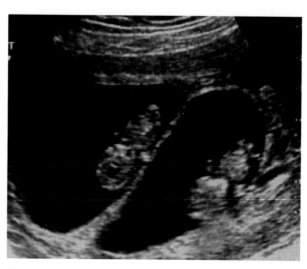

Figure 9.13 Dichorionic twin pregnancy will result in a separate placenta for each fetus. Twin peak sign indicates two separate abutting placentas on the same uterine wall.

Threatened Miscarriage

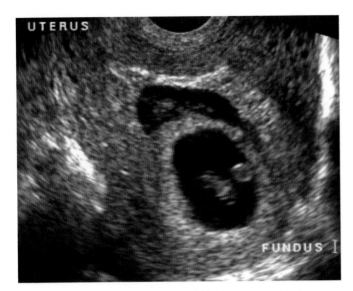

Figure 9.14 Threatened miscarriage with bleeding seen outside the chorionic cavity; however, there is a positive heartbeat.
Courtesy of A Shepherd, Randwick Medical Imaging

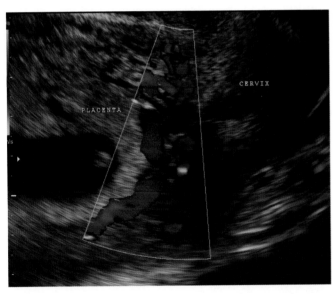

Figure 9.15 Nine-week gestation shows low lying placenta in a patient who presented with bleeding.

A threatened miscarriage is seen as a gestation sac with a fetus and positive heartbeat; however, there is separation of the chorion and a fluid collection (blood) seen. Usually the pregnancy continues and the bleeding resolves.

When the fetus is seen with no fetal heart beat the result is an inevitable miscarriage.

An anembryonic pregnancy occurs when the gestation sac is seen in the uterine cavity but no fetal pole can be identified.

Non-progressive Pregnancy

A miscarriage is the loss of a pregnancy prior to 20–22 weeks' gestation. There are several types including threatened, inevitable, incomplete and complete miscarriage. Other types of pregnancy loss may be due to anembryonic pregnancy, ectopic or molar pregnancy.

When patients present with small uterine size, bleeding or abdominal pain, ultrasound is a valuable tool to assess viability of the pregnancy. The gestation sac should be seen in the body of the uterus.

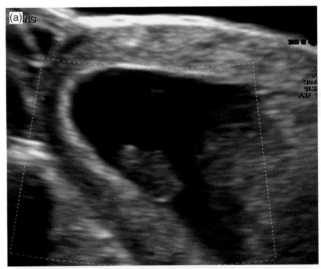

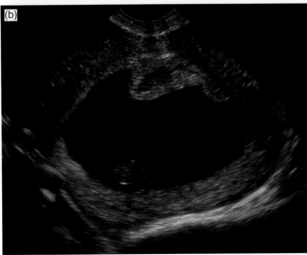

Figure 9.16 Gestational age 11 weeks 4 days with the fetal pole measuring 7 weeks 6 days and no fetal heart movement seen. The transvaginal scan shows an irregular placenta with disproportion between the sac size and the fetal pole.
Courtesy of A Shepherd, Randwick Medical Imaging

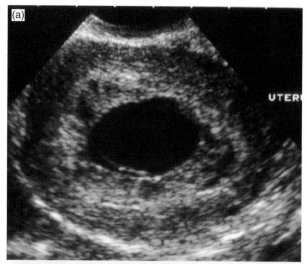

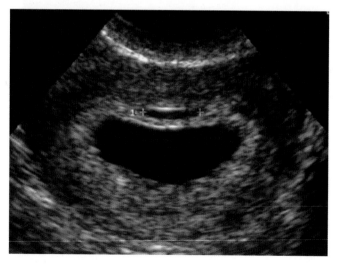

Figure 9.17 Transverse and longitudinal views of an anembryonic gestation.

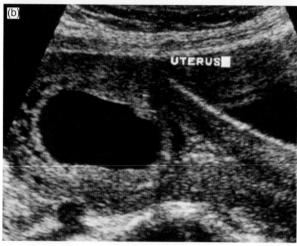

Figure 9.18 Anembryonic non-progressive pregnancy.
Courtesy of A Shepherd, Randwick Medical Imaging

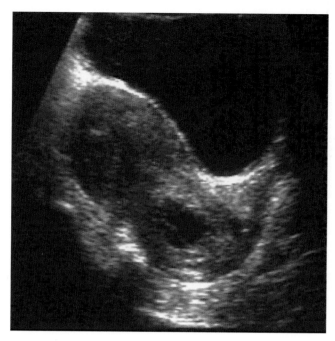

Figure 9.19 In this image the gestation sac is seen in the cervix and resulted in an inevitable miscarriage.

Hydatidiform Mole

A hydatidiform mole or molar pregnancy occurs when the cells that normally form a placenta are replaced by grossly dilated, hydropic villi. This solid collection of echoes is seen on ultrasound with multiple anechoic spaces throughout. No fetal pole develops. Multiple theca luteal cysts may be seen within the ovaries.

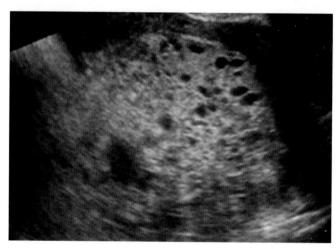

Figure 9.20 Hydatidiform mole.

A partial mole occurs when a normal ovum is fertilised by two sperm, triploid karyotype. The fetus develops, however, with an abnormal karyotype and it cannot survive. Ultrasound will demonstrate focal, hydropic degeneration of the placental villi interspersed with normal placental tissue.

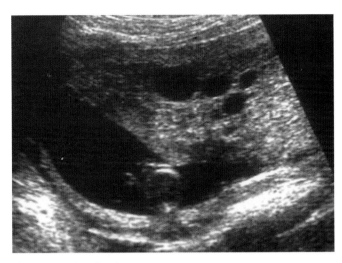

Figure 9.21 Partial mole.

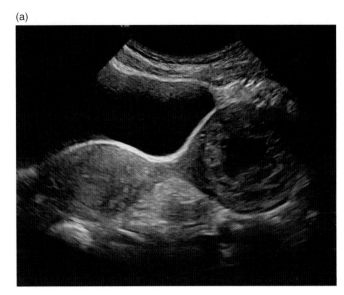

(a)

Ectopic Pregnancy

When no gestation sac can be seen in the uterine cavity and the woman has a positive pregnancy test, further ultrasound investigation of the pelvic region is essential to find or exclude an ectopic implantation.

The majority of ectopic pregnancies occur in the outer part of fallopian tubes, the ampulla. Less often they occur in the isthmus, the inner or narrow segment of the tube. Even less common are interstitial or intramural pregnancy, Caesarean scar implantation, cervical and ovarian pregnancies.

Transabdominal scanning requires a full bladder, to push the bowel up out of the pelvis, to best see the adnexa. The broad ligament may appear thickened on the side of the tubal ectopic implantation.

Transvaginal ultrasound is sensitive enough to show the uterine cavity endometrium and no gestation sac within, free fluid (blood) in the abdominal cavity and the presence of a gestational sac, or a mass in the adnexa.

Definitive diagnosis is when a fetus and fetal heart beat are seen in an ectopic pregnancy. If not treated, the trophoblastic cells will keep growing and rupture the tube, usually with considerable bleeding, resulting in a surgical emergency.

Interstitial or intramural location of an ectopic pregnancy is the most dangerous, as considerable growth is supported by the surrounding tissue of the uterus. These are the least common and require careful transvaginal scanning. Follow the line of the endometrium to the cornu and with manipulation of the beam track the canal through the myometrium, to the gestation sac. Image the gestation sac with the fundal endometrium demonstrating the 'gap' of separation.

Ectopic pregnancies can be hard to diagnose in any location. Heterotopic pregnancies are an intrauterine and an ectopic pregnancy occurring at the same time. Try to manipulate the probe to demonstrate both the intrauterine gestation and the ectopic gestation in one image.

(b)

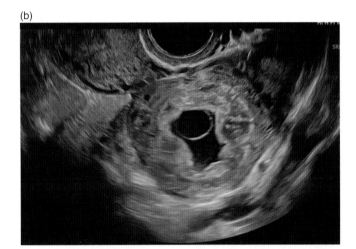

(c)

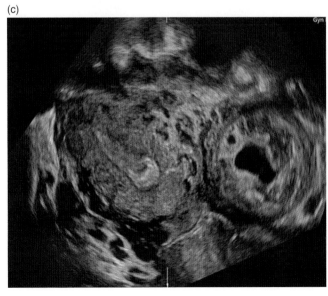

Figure 9.22 (a) Transabdominal transverse view of uterus and the left tubal ectopic gestation. (b) TV scan. Ectopic gestation sac with the yolk sac. (c) Ectopic gestation seen lateral to the uterus using GE OmniView.
Courtesy of R Gibson, Ultrasound Care

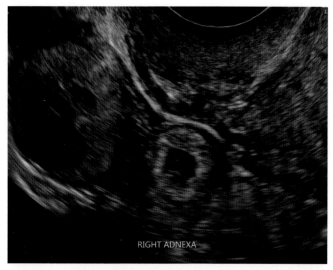

Figure 9.23 Heterotopic pregnancy is an intrauterine and an ectopic pregnancy occurring at the same time. This image shows the corpus luteum on the right and the tubal ectopic. The intrauterine pregnancy is not shown in this image. Courtesy of R Gibson, Ultrasound Care

(a)

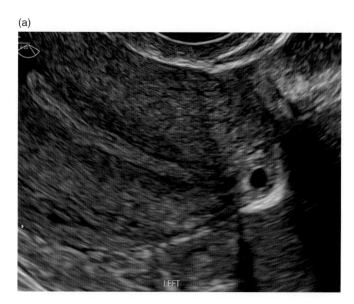

(b)

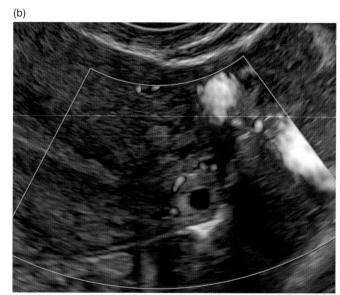

Figure 9.24 (a) Interstitial pregnancy showing the separation of the gestation sac from the fundal endometrium. (b) Interstitial pregnancy. Courtesy of R Gibson, Ultrasound Care

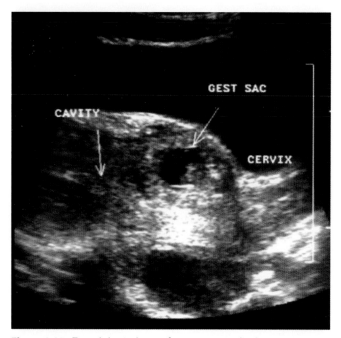

Figure 9.25 Transabdominal scan of a pregnancy in the Caesarean scar.

Why can ectopic pregnancies be missed with ultrasound study?
- Always check for an intrauterine pregnancy first
- Not looking carefully for evidence of a "mass" in the adnexa
- Gestation sac less than 5 weeks' size
- Inadequate depth examined
- Pseudo sac in uterus
- Not extending the examination to check for free fluid in the upper abdomen
- Failure to recognise haemorrhage
- Cervical pregnancy vs. miscarriage
- Poor machine settings
- Inexperience and poor supervision

Chapter

10

Ergonomics

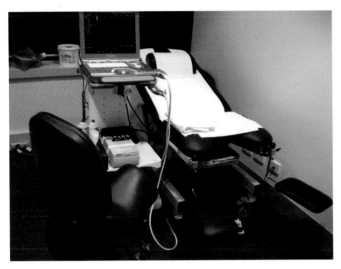

Figure 10.1 The ultrasound console, the couch and the chair are adjusted to individual needs. Being aware of posture will help prevent injury for sonographers.

Sonographers are at risk of injury to the shoulders, neck and back. It is important to be aware of your posture when scanning and not to place repetitive strain on the body. Sonographers need to practice good ergonomics to prevent injury. Stretching and exercise will help reduce the risk of injury.

Ergonomically designed equipment provides for adjustments to the position of the console, bed and chair position, to maintain good posture while scanning.

The machines are designed with height adjustment. If possible, the monitor should be at eye level. The bed can be raised or lowered to suit the individual sonographer.

There are a variety of ergonomically designed chairs.

When scanning, position the ultrasound machine close, so as not to have to reach to operate the console.

Clean and prepare the room before each patient so that the required paper towels, tissues, sheets, gel, etc. are available and within easy access.

Stretching and gentle exercise are recommended to maintain health and prevent injury for sonographers.

Ultrasound has had a positive impact on the management of gynaecology patients and will continue to be a valuable imaging tool in trained hands.

Take care of yourself and enjoy scanning.

Glossary

Acoustic coupling — water, oil or gel is used to remove air between the transduce and the skin for transmission of the ultrasound beam

Acoustic window — moving the probe to maintain an area through which sound can penetrate to visualise deeper structures

Anechoic — echo free, no energy is reflected through fluid filled structures which appear black in an ultrasound image

Artifacts — acoustic artifacts result from the way the ultrasound beam interacts with tissue, causing a range of echogram appearances that do not correspond to anatomical features

Attenuation — loss of energy as the sound beam propagates through tissue

Beam width — slice thickness of detected echoes arising from a three-dimensional volume of tissue and presented in a two-dimensional image

Echogenic — the echoes displayed are brighter compared to the less echogenic or hypoechoic echoes

Enhancement — acoustic enhancement is seen posterior to a non-attenuating fluid filled structure, i.e. enhancement posterior to a cyst

Field of view — the size of the area of tissue seen in one image

Focus — where the beam is narrowest and the focal zone can be adjusted throughout the examination

Freeze — activated so the image will appear in 'Real-time' or to freeze the image to document a still image

Gain — adjusts the overall amplification of the echoes

Hyperechoic — more echogenic (whiter) echoes

Hypoechoic — less echogenic (darker) echoes

Real-time — automatic rapid repeat of the scan action producing an ultrasound image updated many times a second

Shadow — acoustic shadowing is seen posterior to a strongly attenuating interface i.e. between soft tissue and bone or air or other strongly attenuating tissue

Time Gain Compensation (TGC) — TGC echoes from deeper tissues are more attenuated and can be amplified, using the TGC to ensure even shades of grey, to produce a uniform tissue appearance

References

Australian Society for Ultrasound in Medicine. Standards of practice. Available at: www.asum.com.au

Baird DD, Dunson DB, Hill MC, Cousins D, Schectman JM. High cumulative incidence of uterine leiomyoma in black and white women: ultrasound evidence. *Am J Obstet Gynecol* 2003;**188**(1):100–7.

Basseal J and van de Mortel TF. Guidelines for reprocessing ultrasound transducers. *Austral J Ultrasound Medi* 2017;**20**:30–40.

Brohl AS, Li L, Andikyan V, et al. Age-stratified risk of unexpected uterine sarcoma following surgery for presumed benign leiomyoma. *Oncologist* 2015;**20**(4):433–9.

Callen, P. Ultrasound in obstetrics and gynecology. WB Saunders, 1994.

Casini ML, Rossi F, Agostini R, Unfer V. Effects of the position of fibroids on fertility. *Gynecol Oncol* 2006;**22**(2):106–9.

Dreisler E, Stampe Sorensen S, Ibsen PH, Lose G. Prevalence of endometrial polyps and abnormal uterine bleeding in a Danish population aged 20–74 years. *Ultrasound Obstet Gynecol* 2009;**33**(1):102–8.

Gent R. Applied physics and technology of diagnostic ultrasound. Milner Publishing, 1997.

Gill R. The physics and technology of diagnostic ultrasound: a practitioner's guide. High Frequency Publishing, 2012.

Jansen, R. Getting pregnant. Allen & Unwin, 2003.

Kumar V, Cotran, R, Robbins, S. Basic pathology. WB Saunders, 1992.

Lee SC, Kaunitz AM, Sanchez-Ramos L, Rhatigan RM. The oncogenic potential of endometrial polyps: a systematic review and meta-analysis. *Obstet Gynaecol* 2010;**116**(5):1197–1205.

Llewellyn-Jones D. Fundamentals of obstetrics and gynaecology, 4th ed., Vol. 2. The Chaucer Press, 1986.

Menakaya U, Reid S, Infante F, Condous G. Systematic evaluation of women with suspected endometriosis using a 5-domain sonographically based approach. *J Ultrasound Med* 2015;**34**:937–47.

Moore LK, Dalley AF, Agur AMR. Clinically oriented anatomy, 7th ed. Lippincott Williams & Wilkins, 2014.

Munro MG, Critchley HOD, Broder MS, Fraser IS. FIGO classification system (PALM-COEIN) for causes of abnormal uterine bleeding in nongravid women of reproductive age. *Int J Gynecol Obstet* 2011;**113**:3–13.

Naji O, Abdallah Y, Bij De Vaate AJ, et al. Standardized approach for imaging and measuring Cesarean section scars using ultrasonography. *Ultrasound Obstet Gynecol* 2012;**39**:252–9.

Perez-Medina T, Bajo-Arenas J, Salazar F, Redondo T, Sanfrutos L, Alvarez P, Engels V. Endometrial polyps and their implication in the pregnancy rates of patients undergoing intrauterine insemination: a prospective, randomized study. *Hum Reprod* 2005;**20**(6):1632–5.

Practice Committee of the American Society for Reproductive Medicine. Removal of myomas in asymptomatic patients to improve fertility and/or reduce miscarriage rate: a guideline. *Fertil Steril* 2017;**108**(3):416–25.

Sherwood L. Human physiology: from cells to systems, 4th ed. Brooks/Cole, 2001.

Index